Healthy Cooking

WITH ESSENTIAL OIL

Healthy Cooking
with Essential Oil

Rebecca Park Totilo

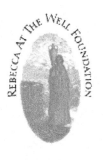

Healthy Cooking with Essential Oil

ISBN 978-0-9898280-4-8

Table of Contents

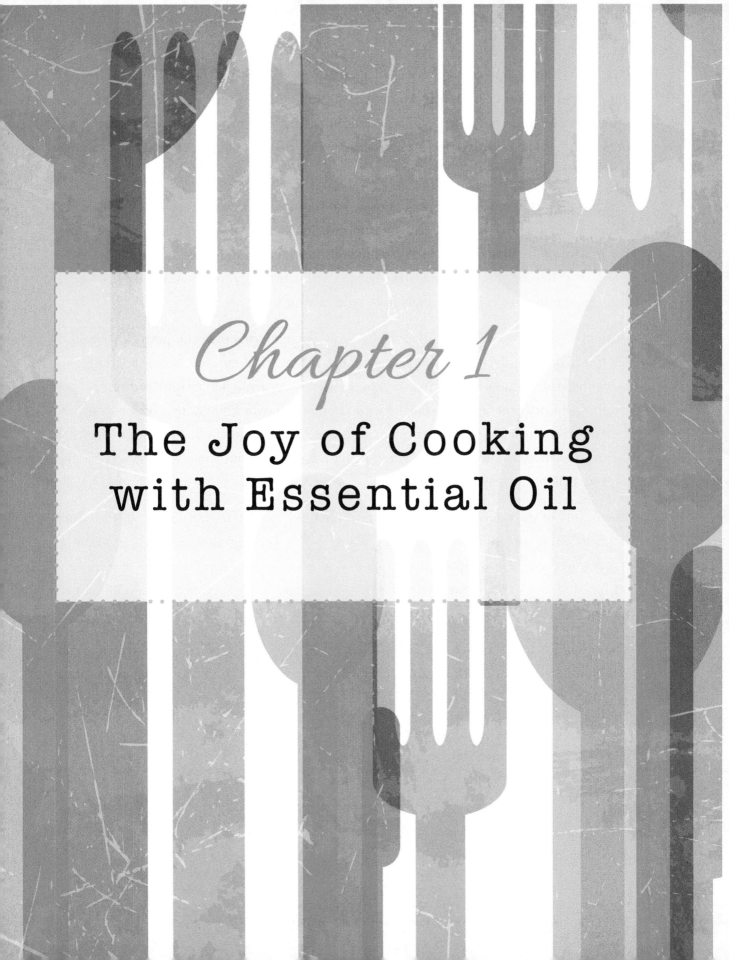

Chapter 1
The Joy of Cooking with Essential Oil

Can you imagine opening the doors to a whole new world of cooking, unleashing new dimensions of sensory pleasure? Aromatherapy can enhance your culinary creations in a multitude of ways, using essential oils to add more than just fragrance or flavor. Food is not merely fuel; it can be enjoyed as a multi-sensory experience that brings therapeutic value as well as nourishment.

The virtues of essential oils are well known, but their benefits extend beyond the treatment room. Cooking with essential oils can open up a wealth of creative opportunities in the kitchen. For years we have limited the use of essential oils to scented candles and massage oils, in the belief that they are unsafe to consume. But the tide is turning – more and more people are realizing the value of using essential oils to enhance our food.

Ancient civilizations recognized this a long time ago, understanding the power of essential oils to add depth and flavor to their food. Modern society lost these ancient cookery traditions as synthetic substitutes became more popular. Recent generations have missed out on the amazing sensory experience of cooking with essential oils, which not only produces delicious creations but also enhances the entire cooking process from start to finish. Just one or two drops can transform your kitchen into a fragrant paradise, filled with mouth-watering aromatic treats to delight the senses.

The beauty of essential oils is that only a tiny amount is needed to transform your dish from rather plain to something truly amazing. Being highly concentrated, every drop is a little powerhouse of flavor and packed with natural goodness. From condiments to desserts and drinks, almost any recipe can be enhanced with the right oil – experimentation is all part of the fun!

The aroma of food can account for as much as 90% of its perceived flavor. Essential oils can be used to add aromatic depth, providing new flavors that can be as strong or as subtle

Because essential oils are so highly concentrated, they are 50 to 70 times more therapeutically potent than the herbs or plants they are derived from. Dried herbs lose up to 90% of their healing nutrients and oxygen molecules, whereas essential oils do not.

as desired. Think of it as just another way of adding seasoning to your food, like herbs and spices.

But essential oils offer more than just fragrance and flavor – their therapeutic qualities can actually help to improve your overall wellbeing, as well as making your food taste delicious. Unlike other cooking oils, essential oils are fat-free.

Salad dressings, dips and marinades are good places to start for beginners. A drop of an herbal essential oil can replace around one tablespoon of fresh herbs as a general guideline. You will be amazed at the powerful flavors that such a tiny amount of essential oil can add to a recipe – the merest hint is sometimes all it takes to really add the 'wow factor' to a dish. Your dinner guests will love the sensory experience!

You might still feel uneasy about consuming essential oils – after all, it goes against our instincts to drink substances that we are led to believe are toxic. But if you chew gum or use toothpaste it is likely that you have already consumed essential oils without realizing it, as they are commonly used in the confectionery industry to add flavor. And if you've enjoyed a glass of Coca-Cola recently, you might be interested to learn that its secret recipe contains 16 different essential oils, including vanilla, cinnamon, orange and lime.

The FDA has published an extensive list of essential oils that are safe to consume in small doses. While some do contain toxic components, the miniscule amounts used in cooking render them to be harmless. Many common store-cupboard ingredients are toxic at high doses but considered to be safe in moderation – such as salt, which is found in almost every kitchen. As long as you are using pure therapeutic quality oils, you can rest assured that they are suitable for consumption.

Aromatherapy harnesses the wonderful natural power of essential oils, so incorporating them into your everyday cooking is a great way to enjoy their therapeutic properties. The act of cooking itself will be enhanced by the fragrant pleasure of adding essential oils, soothing the

Taking essential oils internally is more commonplace in France, where physicians often prescribe therapeutic-grade oils to treat a range of physical disorders. They have been proven to help boost immunity, improve circulation, neutralize toxins and purify the internal systems of the body.

mind or reinvigorating the senses. What could be more enjoyable than spending time in the kitchen surrounded by wonderful aromas, creating delicious food for you and your loved ones?

Many people are unfamiliar with essential oils or unsure how to use them safely in cookery. This guide is designed to demystify the concept of adding essential oils to food, hopefully inspiring you to leap into the kitchen and begin experimenting to create your own aromatic delights! The opportunities are truly endless. If you have been missing out on this wonderful sensory experience it's time to get cooking!

"When you use essential oils in the kitchen, there is no end to the interesting tastes you can create"

– Valerie Ann Worwood,
Aromatherapist and author of
The Complete Book of Essential Oils and Aromatherapy

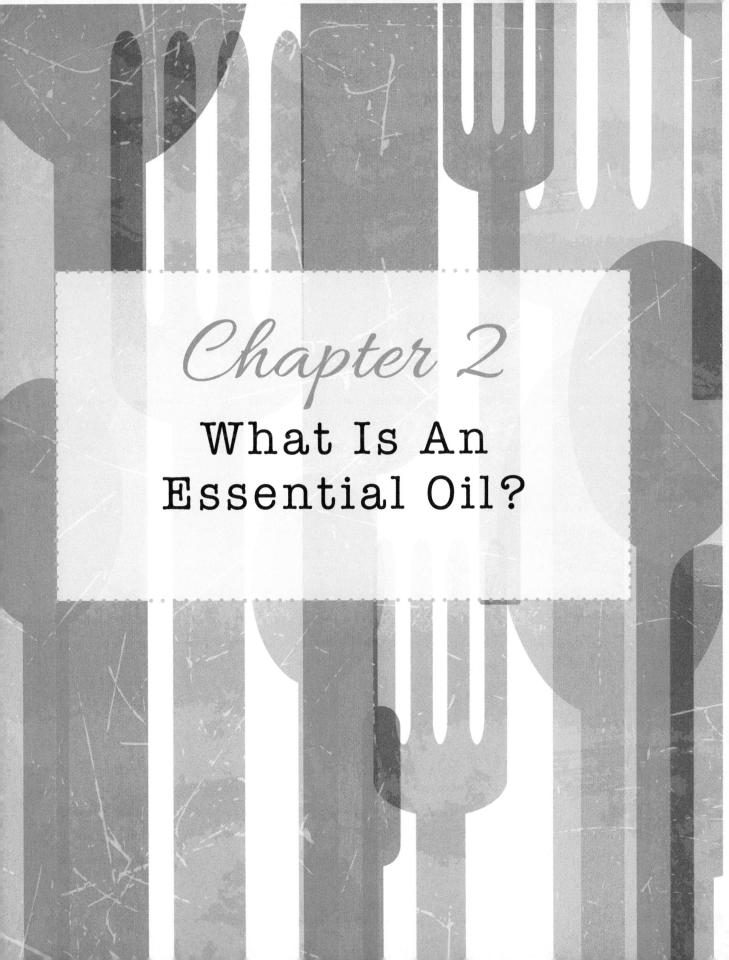

Chapter 2
What Is An Essential Oil?

Essential oils are fragrant, vital fluids distilled from flowers, shrubs, leaves, trees, roots, and seeds. Technically, they are actually not "oil" at all, but are volatile organic compounds made up of a variety of chemicals.

Before adding an essential oil in a favorite casserole or dish, you will need to understand what essential oils are, as well as learn about their unique aroma and characteristics. Study their aroma profiles so you will know which ones to use to enhance your recipe.

ESSENTIAL OIL VS. VEGETABLE OIL

Since essential oils are derived from a natural plant source, you will notice that the oil does not leave an "oily" or greasy spot. This is because essential oils do not contain any lipids, unlike fatty vegetable oils used in cooking, such as olive, flax, coconut, avocado, or canola. Vegetable oils, on the other hand, are 100% fat and contain glycerol, which leaves a greasy residue. Vegetable oils are important to our health as well, as they contain fatty acids essential for bodily functions that the body cannot produce on its own.

While both essential oils and vegetable oils have many health benefits, essential oils offer a holistic alternative to vegetable oils in many ways:

- Essential oils' unique chemistry makeup enables them to be able to permeate every cell and administer healing at the most fundamental level of our body.
- Essential oils' structural complexity enables them to perform various functions with just a few drops of oil. Essential oils are steam distilled from plants (with the exception of citrus oils which are cold-pressed).

ESSENTIAL OIL VS. DRIED HERBS

Essential oils are extremely concentrated with more intense flavor – more than 50 to 70 times more potent than the fresh or dried herb they are derived from! Because of their potency, you will never want to add more than a drop or two at a time to a recipe (unless the recipe instructs otherwise). In comparison to dried herbs, adding 1/2 teaspoon to a recipe is quite common and may not seem like much, however, with essential oils a teaspoon is approximately 76 drops, which is quite a lot. In fact, just one drop of peppermint oil is equivalent to approximately 28 cups of tea. And when you consider it only takes a few leaves of peppermint to make tea, it takes five pounds of leaves to make one ounce of essential oil.

You will find that having essential oils on hand in your kitchen pantry is just as convenient as dried herbs and can be great for longer cooking times.

While both essential oils and fresh and dried herbs add flavor and aroma to an entrée, essential oils do offer additional benefits:

> Essential oils are distilled from various parts of the plant including leaves, flowers, roots, seeds, bark, resins, or expressed from the rinds of citrus fruits. It normally takes at least 50 pounds of plant material to make one pound of essential oil. For example, a pound of rosemary oil requires sixty-six pounds of herbs.

- Dried herbs lose up to 90% of their healing nutrients, whereas essential oils' healing constituents remain intact. Essential oils contain virtually all of the plant's healing nutrients, including oxygenating molecules, amino acid precursors, coenzyme A factors, trace minerals, enzymes, vitamins, hormones and more.

- Dried herbs contain only 3-5% of their essential oil after the drying process, which means they do not give off the aroma or flavor as an essential oil of the same plant. With essential oils, you receive all of the great taste of traditional herbs and spices without preservatives.

- Essential oils are 50 to 70 times more therapeutically potent than the herbs or plants they are derived from.

- Essential oils have a longer shelf life than dried herbs and don't go stale like dried herbs. Essential oils keep their intense flavor for years.

While certain essential oils can be harmful if used in high dosages, moderate use for flavoring a favorite dish is not only safe but scrumptious! Essential oils can be the star of a dish or they can add subtle layers of flavor which highlight other ingredients.

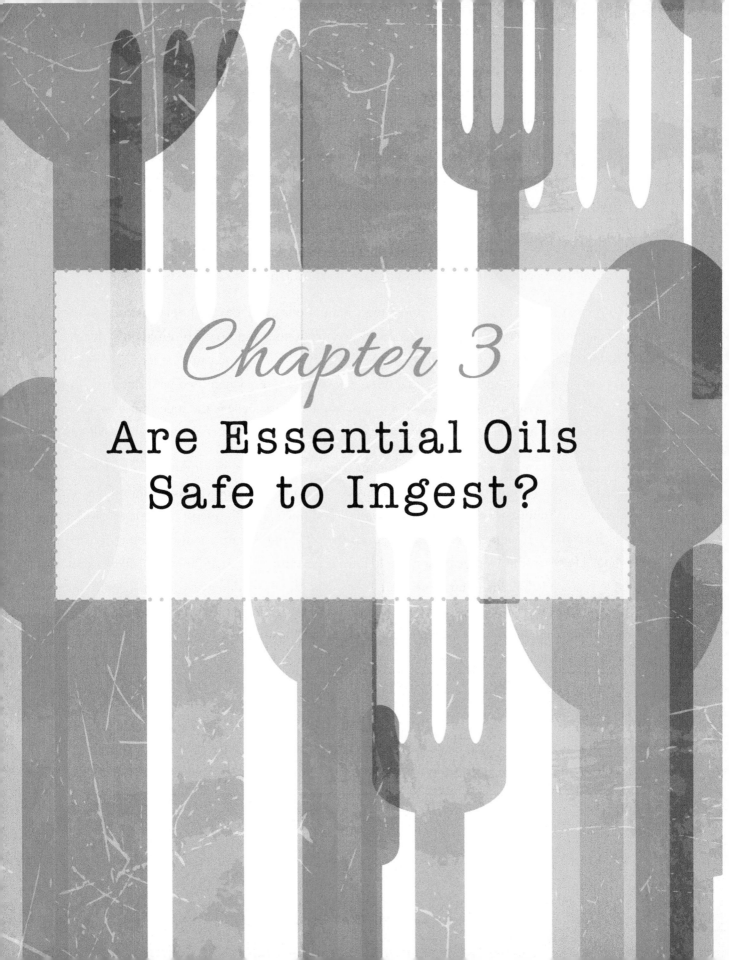

Chapter 3

Are Essential Oils Safe to Ingest?

For years we have avoided taking essential oils internally in the belief that they are toxic substances and dangerous to consume. Society has accepted the use of essential oils in skin care products, but is yet to embrace the potential advantages of adding them to our food.

The concept of ingesting essential oils is nothing new – evidence has shown that this was common practice throughout ancient civilizations. The majority of modern aromatherapy advice warns against ever consuming essential oils, claiming that they should only be used externally and in diluted form. It is, therefore, no wonder that most people have never considered using essential oils in cookery. The fear of the unknown has prevented essential oils from being considered as valid ingredients in the kitchen.

However, most of us are already ingesting essential oils every day without realizing, as they are commonly used to add flavoring in the confectionery industry. Hundreds of everyday products, such as toothpaste and cola, rely on essential oils for their unique flavor. This only serves to prove that ingesting essential oils is not toxic per se – when used with due care, they can be a wonderful addition to our daily diet. Some experts believe the ingestion of essential oils is not only harmless, but can be positively beneficial to our internal health and wellbeing.

The beauty of adding essential oils to your food is that only a tiny quantity is required to inject a huge amount of flavor. Yes, essential oils do contain some toxic components, but when using minuscule amounts they are rendered harmless. Nutmeg is known to produce psychotropic and hallucinogenic effects, with the potential to cause acute poisoning if eaten whole. However, the average person would have to consume at least 100ml of nutmeg essential oil to reach a lethal dose – far more than would ever be required in everyday cookery. In fact, the amount of essential oils that would be required to produce a toxic effect would result in food so unpalatable that we would instinctively avoid consuming it.

Tip:
Dr. Phillip Minton states, "Eating pure essential oils can improve circulation and oxygenation and protect against heart disease, dementia and cancer."

HOW ESSENTIAL OILS ARE METABOLIZED BY THE BODY

While ingesting essential oils through the oral route, care should be taken due to the potential toxicity of some essential oils. Essential oil compounds and their metabolites that are ingested are absorbed in the digestive tract and enter the blood stream where they are distributed to their target organs.

It is confirmed by various research findings that essential oils are rapidly absorbed into the blood stream after administration through dermal, oral or pulmonary (via inhalation) route. They then cross the blood-brain barrier and attach to the various receptors present in the central nervous system and produce their effects of improving sleep, relaxing the mind and body, benefiting digestion, and more.

It has also been confirmed in studies that the majority of the components in essential oils metabolized in the body are either eliminated or excreted by the kidneys, or exhaled by the lungs in the form of carbon dioxide. It is believed that there is minimum risk of accumulation of essential oils in the body tissues because the active compounds present in them are metabolized quickly and have a short half-life.

TOXICITY OF ESSENTIAL OILS

Certain essential oils could have irritation potential and can be toxic if large doses are ingested. For this reason, only a drop or two is used in cooking.

Some of the short-term complications of ingesting essential oils in large doses are:

- Essential oils may cause burning of the mucous membranes of the oral cavity, throat and esophagus.
- Essential oils may also lead to occurrence of reflux by irritating the digestive tract.
- Certain essential oils may cause symptoms of nausea, vomiting and/or diarrhea.
- Essential oils may also interfere with certain medications and can make them useless or lead to complications such as seizures.
- Essential oils also have the potential to interfere with anesthesia.
- Essential oils can elevate the liver enzymes.

Some of the long-term complications of ingesting essential oils are: Ingesting essential oils long term can cause liver cancer, liver failure, enlargement of liver, and fatty liver disease (all of these complications occur due to undue stress on the liver by metabolizing the essential oils), and kidney failure.

Tip:

Daniel Pénoël, M.D. recommends using essential oils in food preparation as they purify the body, enhance the immune system and generate endorphins.

HOW ARE ESSENTIAL OILS EXCRETED FROM THE BODY?

When essential oils are applied topically or inhaled, they initially bypass the liver and interact with the target organs to produce their desired effect. Finally, the essential oils metabolites enter the blood and lymph, are redirected to the liver and ultimately excreted via the intestinal and urinary tract.

In the case of oral ingestion of essential oils, they are absorbed into the blood stream and directed to the liver by the time they have reached the small intestine. In the liver the essential oil molecules are metabolized to form various phytochemicals which are further broken down. The essential oil can become toxic when the liver prefers to metabolize other substances first, instead of the essential oil phytochemicals. This can lead to accumulation of the phytochemicals in the liver. These phytochemicals can sometimes reach toxic amounts. For instance, a common bioactive fraction of peppermint oil, 1,8 cineole, is not preferred by the liver and it can quickly accumulate to dangerous levels causing liver failure.

Different protocols exist for ingesting essential oils orally. This largely depends on the body part to which the action of essential oil is targeted. You should be aware of these protocols before ingesting essential oils orally.

Be sure to exercise caution if you are taking any medications, as their interaction with essential oil components may hinder their effectiveness. If in doubt, consult a qualified Aromatherapist for advice.

Essential oils can be quite effective if the proper protocol is followed when you are ingesting them orally. Take care to be aware of the dosage, the effects and potential toxicity of the particular essential oil you are planning to ingest orally or use in cooking. If taken in small doses (preferably a couple of drops initially), essential oils can be used effectively to relieve many physical and emotional health issues or enhance your cooking.

Essential oils are not water-soluble but are made water-soluble by various enzymes found in the liver. From there, they are excreted by the kidneys via urine. When an essential oil component is introduced to the body at a faster rate than the liver can convert it into a water-soluble form, liver toxicity can result. (This can happen from any mode of entry, not just ingestion.)

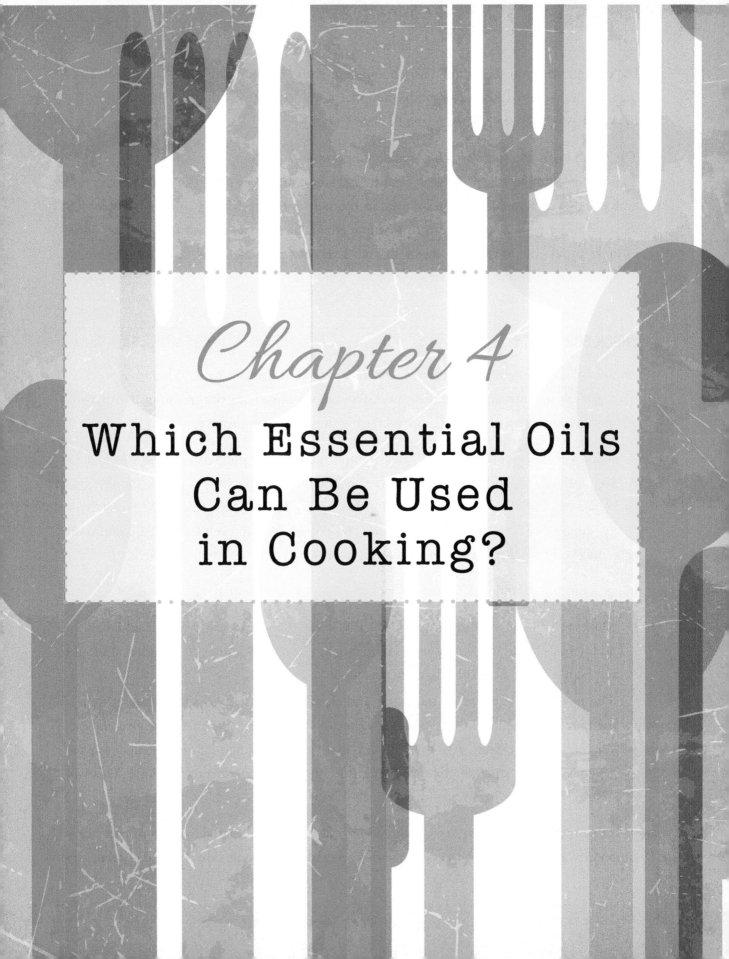

Chapter 4

Which Essential Oils Can Be Used in Cooking?

For internal use, you should only use therapeutic-grade oils that are 100% pure, preferably organic, and sourced from a reputable supplier. Only choose oils that are included on the FDA's GRAS ("Generally Recognized As Safe") list.

The second consideration, which is equally important, is to check the quality of the oil. The majority of essential oils available at health food stores and especially those sold at bath and body shops are manufactured to be used in the perfume industry. It is highly possible that these oils have been adulterated with multiple chemicals so as to extend the essential oil or to make an alteration in the scent of the oil. Even the oils tagged as natural may contain contaminants and there is no guarantee of its purity.

CHECK FOR PURITY

Always try to use essential oils from a reliable source that you can trust. Whenever possible, purchase oils that are organic and steam distilled at very low temperatures to insure that the oil's constituents have not been destroyed during the distillation process.

Sometimes it is difficult to know if the essential oil you are purchasing is of the highest grade. One way to find out is to contact the essential oil company and ask for the Gas Chromatography/Mass Spectrometry (GC-MS) report. This analysis assures the buyer of its purity and quality by identifying each of the components within each batch of oil and their percentages. This process also identifies any adulteration of the essential oil tested.

In addition, you should look for the following qualities in an essential oil:

- Make sure that the oil is genuine and it is 100% natural without any synthetic additives. In addition, it should be 100% pure with no other essential oils added into it. The oil should not be recolored, decolorized or deterpenated.
- The essential oil should be authentic and should be from the specific species that is mentioned on the label. It is essential to check for the purity and quality of essential oils you are using internally so as to make sure that you are getting the true benefits from the essential oil and know the oil's characteristics and certain predictable actions. This will ensure you are not ingesting any chemicals with the oils.

As with any chemical, common sense should prevail. Keep in mind that many common store-cupboard ingredients can be toxic in high doses, such as basic table salt. Anything potentially toxic should always be appropriately stored away from children and only used under supervision. Always remember that moderation is the key – adhere to the recommended dosage and dilution guidelines and you should not experience any problems at all. Even some oils that are GRAS certified should be cautiously used. For instance, wintergreen is safe to use as a food additive but it is not recommended to ingest the oil orally.

There are several essential oils that should never be taken internally, including camphor, citronella, thuja, pennyroyal, sassafras, wormseed and wormwood.

GRAS FL AND FA ESSENTIAL OILS

According to the FDA (Food and Drug Administration) the following essential oils, oleoresins (CO2), and natural extractives including distillates are listed as GRAS (Generally Regarded As Safe) for their intended use, according to section 108.20 of the Code of Regulations and section 409 of the Act. FA is designation for ingredients that are approved as food additives. Most of the essential oils on this list are classified as FA, as many are used for food flavorings and preservatives (due to their high antioxidant capability and antimicrobial actions).

Essential oils on the FDA GRAS list are considered safe for human consumption. Many on this list, however, have not been tested by current methods and have been grandfathered into use by virtue of being widely used in the food industry for several decades without any reported negative effects.

Most essential oils on this list are safe for ingestion in amounts commonly prescribed in medical aromatherapy protocols. These amounts are VERY small which does not imply they are safe at any dosage. Please be aware of the safety considerations and the recommended amounts covered in this book.

Tip:

Only use pure essential oils that are on the FDA GRAS and FA list. Oils not listed are probably not safe for ingestion. If unsure, do not use in cooking.

What the FDA GRAS list does not provide is recommended dosages that are considered safe. The FDA's documentation does note that items on the list are safe in commonly used amounts, or amounts adequate to accomplish the necessary effect as a food additive. For essential oils, this means approximate doses in the range of 1 to 3 drops, 1 to 3 times per day. These are the amounts noted in most clinical or medical aromatherapy protocols. Even still, there are essential oils on the GRAS list that should be used with caution or not at all for ingestion, particularly by individuals who have certain medical conditions, or are pregnant or lactating. When using essential oils in cooking or for ingestion, it is crucial for your safety that you are following a protocol appropriate for your health. You will want to make sure you know what the appropriate dosages should be. When in doubt, seek the guidance of a qualified health professional before proceeding with ingesting essential oils.

Not all essential oils that are on the FDA's GRAS list are recommended for ingestion – take for instance, wintergreen. While it is considered a safe food additive, the commonly used amount as a food additive is considerably small, and even a drop or two of this oil is significantly greater than the amount in a piece of chewing gum, for example.

ESSENTIAL OILS GRAS LIST

Essential oils, oleoresins (solvent-free), and natural extractives (including distillates) that are generally recognized as safe for their intended use, within the meaning of section 409 of the Act, are as follows:

Common Name	Botanical Name (plant source)
Alfalfa	Medicago sativa L.
Allspice	Pimenta officinalis Lindl.
Almond, bitter (free from prussic acid)	Prunus amygdalus Batsch, Prunus armeniaca L., or Prunus persica (L.) Batsch.
Ambrette (seed)	Hibiscus moschatus Moench.
Angelica root	Angelica archangelica L.
Angelica seed	Do.
Angelica stem	Do.
Angostura (cusparia bark)	Galipea officinalis Hancock.
Anise	Pimpinella anisum L.
Asafetida	Ferula assa-foetida L. and related spp. of Ferula.
Balm (lemon balm)	Melissa officinalis L.
Balsam of Peru	Myroxylon pereirae Klotzsch.
Basil	Ocimum basilicum L.
Bay leaves	Laurus nobilis L.
Bay (myrcia oil)	Pimenta racemosa (Mill.) J. W. Moore.
Bergamot (bergamot orange)	Citrus aurantium L. subsp. bergamia Wright et Arn.
Bitter almond (free from prussic acid)	Prunus amygdalus Batsch, Prunus armeniaca L., or Prunus persica (L.) Batsch.
Bois de rose	Aniba rosaeodora Ducke.
Cacao	Theobroma cacao L.
Camomile (chamomile) flowers, Hungarian	Matricaria chamomilla L.
Camomile (chamomile) flowers, Roman or English	Anthemis nobilis L.
Cananga	Cananga odorata Hook. f. and Thoms.
Capsicum	Capsicum frutescens L. and Capsicum annuum L.
Caraway	Carum carvi L.
Cardamom seed (cardamon)	Elettaria cardamomum Maton.
Carob bean	Ceratonia siliqua L.
Carrot	Daucus carota L.
Cascarilla bark	Croton eluteria Benn.
Cassia bark, Chinese	Cinnamomum cassia Blume.
Cassia bark, Padang or Batavia	Cinnamomum burmanni Blume.
Cassia bark, Saigon	Cinnamomum loureirii Nees.
Celery seed	Apium graveolens L.

Common Name	Botanical Name (plant source)
Cherry, wild, bark	Prunus serotina Ehrh.
Chervil	Anthriscus cerefolium (L.) Hoffm.
Chicory	Cichorium intybus L.
Cinnamon bark, Ceylon	Cinnamomum zeylanicum Nees.
Cinnamon bark, Chinese	Cinnamomum cassia Blume.
Cinnamon bark, Saigon	Cinnamomum loureirii Nees.
Cinnamon leaf, Ceylon	Cinnamomum zeylanicum Nees.
Cinnamon leaf, Chinese	Cinnamomum cassia Blume.
Cinnamon leaf, Saigon	Cinnamomum loureirii Nees.
Citronella	Cymbopogon nardus Rendle.
Citrus peels	Citrus spp.
Clary (clary sage)	Salvia sclarea L.
Clover	Trifolium spp.
Coca (decocainized)	Erythroxylum coca Lam. and other spp. of Erythroxylum.
Coffee	Coffea spp.
Cola nut	Cola acuminata Schott and Endl., and other spp. of Cola.
Coriander	Coriandrum sativum L.
Cumin (cummin)	Cuminum cyminum L.
Curacao orange peel (orange, bitter peel)	Citrus aurantium L.
Cusparia bark	Galipea officinalis Hancock.
Dandelion	Taraxacum officinale Weber and T. laevigatum DC.
Dandelion root	Do.
Dog grass (quackgrass, triticum)	Agropyron repens (L.) Beauv.
Elder flowers	Sambucus canadensis L. and S. nigra l.
Estragole (esdragol, esdragon, tarragon)	Artemisia dracunculus L.
Estragon (tarragon)	Do.
Fennel, sweet	Foeniculum vulgare Mill.
Fenugreek	Trigonella foenum-graecum L.
Galanga (galangal)	Alpinia officinarum Hance.
Geranium	Pelargonium spp.
Geranium, East Indian	Cymbopogon martini Stapf.
Geranium, rose	Pelargonium graveolens L'Her.

Common Name	Botanical Name (plant source)
Ginger	Zingiber officinale Rosc.
Grapefruit	Citrus paradisi Macf.
Guava	Psidium spp.
Hickory bark	Carya spp.
Horehound (hoarhound)	Marrubium vulgare L.
Hops	Humulus lupulus L.
Horsemint	Monarda punctata L.
Hyssop	Hyssopus officinalis L.
Immortelle	Helichrysum augustifolium DC.
Jasmine	Jasminum officinale L. and other spp. of Jasminum.
Juniper (berries)	Juniperus communis L.
Kola nut	Cola acuminata Schott and Endl., and other spp. of Cola.
Laurel berries	Laurus nobilis L.
Laurel leaves	Laurus spp.
Lavender	Lavandula officinalis Chaix.
Lavender, spike	Lavandula latifolia Vill.
Lavandin	Hybrids between Lavandula officinalis Chaix and Lavandula latifolin Vill.
Lemon	Citrus limon (L.) Burm. f.
Lemon balm (see balm)	
Lemon grass	Cymbopogon citratus DC. and Cymbopogon lexuosus Stapf.
Lemon peel	Citrus limon (L.) Burm. f.
Lime	Citrus aurantifolia Swingle.
Linden flowers	Tilia spp.
Locust bean	Ceratonia siliqua L,
Lupulin	Humulus lupulus L.
Mace	Myristica fragrans Houtt.
Mandarin	Citrus reticulata Blanco.
Marjoram, sweet	Majorana hortensis Moench.
Mate	Ilex paraguariensis St. Hil.
Melissa (see balm)	
Menthol	Mentha spp.
Menthyl acetate	Do.
Molasses (extract)	Saccarum officinarum L.

Common Name	Botanical Name (plant source)
Mustard	Brassica spp.
Naringin	Citrus paradisi Macf.
Neroli, bigarade	Citrus aurantium L.
Nutmeg	Myristica fragrans Houtt.
Onion	Allium cepa L.
Orange, bitter, flowers	Citrus aurantium L.
Orange, bitter, peel	Do.
Orange leaf	Citrus sinensis (L.) Osbeck.
Orange, sweet	Do.
Orange, sweet, flowers	Do.
Orange, sweet, peel	Do.
Origanum	Origanum spp.
Palmarosa	Cymbopogon martini Stapf.
Paprika	Capsicum annuum L.
Parsley	Petroselinum crispum (Mill.) Mansf.
Pepper, black	Piper nigrum L.
Pepper, white	Do.
Peppermint	Mentha piperita L.
Peruvian balsam	Myroxylon pereirae Klotzsch.
Petitgrain	Citrus aurantium L.
Petitgrain lemon	Citrus limon (L.) Burm. f.
Petitgrain mandarin or tangerine	Citrus reticulata Blanco.
Pimenta	Pimenta officinalis Lindl.
Pimenta leaf	Pimenta officinalis Lindl.
Pipsissewa leaves	Chimaphila umbellata Nutt.
Pomegranate	Punica granatum L.
Prickly ash bark	Xanthoxylum (or Zanthoxylum) Americanum Mill. or Xanthoxylum clava-herculis L.
Rose absolute	Rosa alba L., Rosa centifolia L., Rosa damascena Mill., Rosa gallica L., and vars. of these spp.
Rose (otto of roses, attar of roses)	Do.
Rose buds	Do.
Rose flowers	Do.
Rose fruit (hips)	Do.
Rose geranium	Pelargonium graveolens L'Her.

Common Name	Botanical Name (plant source)
Rose leaves	Rosa spp.
Rosemary	Rosmarinus officinalis L.
Saffron	Crocus sativus L.
Sage	Salvia officinalis L.
Sage, Greek	Salvia triloba L.
Sage, Spanish	Salvia lavandulaefolia Vahl.
St. John's bread	Ceratonia siliqua L.
Savory, summer	Satureia hortensis L.
Savory, winter	Satureia montana L.
Schinus molle	Schinus molle L.
Sloe berries (blackthorn berries)	Prunus spinosa L.
Spearmint	Mentha spicata L.
Spike lavender	Lavandula latifolia Vill.
Tamarind	Tamarindus indica L.
Tangerine	Citrus reticulata Blanco.
Tarragon	Artemisia dracunculus L.
Tea	Thea sinensis L.
Thyme	Thymus vulgaris L. and Thymus zygis var. gracilis Boiss.
Thyme, white	Do.
Thyme, wild or creeping	Thymus serpyllum L.
Triticum (see dog grass)	
Tuberose	Polianthes tuberosa L.
Turmeric	Curcuma longa L.
Vanilla	Vanilla planifolia Andr. or Vanilla tahitensis J. W. Moore.
Violet flowers	Viola odorata L.
Violet leaves	Do.
Violet leaves absolute	Do.
Wild cherry bark	Prunus serotina Ehrh.
Ylang-ylang	Cananga odorata Hook. f. and Thoms.
Zedoary bark	Curcuma zedoaria Rosc.

[42 FR 14640, Mar. 15, 1977, as amended at 44 FR 3963, Jan. 19, 1979; 47 FR 29953, July 9, 1982; 48 FR 51613, Nov. 10, 1983; 50 FR 21043 and 21044, May 22, 1985]

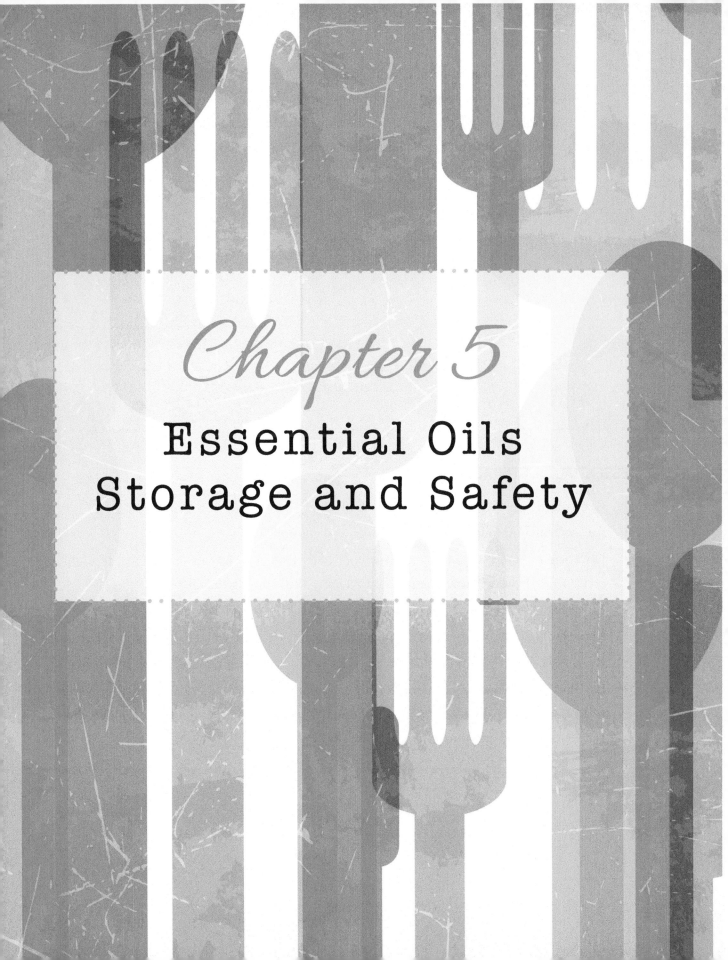

Chapter 5

Essential Oils Storage and Safety

Because essential oils contain no fatty acids, they are not susceptible to rancidity like vegetable oils – but you will want to protect them from the degenerative effects of heat, light, and air. Store them in tightly sealed, dark glass bottles away from any heat source. Properly stored oils can maintain their quality for years. (Citrus oils are less stable and should not be stored longer than six months to a year after opening.)

Rosemary, thyme, sage, and other essential oils can last between 3-4 years. Citrus oils can last 1-2 years when stored properly. One way to preserve your essential oils is to keep them refrigerated. In doing so, they will last twice as long. Be sure to keep them in a lunch cooler, small container or ziplock bag while stored in the refrigerator, since food may start to taste like the essential oils. If you have a large collection of essential oils, you may want to purchase a small student-size fridge that is solely dedicated to your oils.

ESSENTIAL OIL STORAGE:

- Keep oils tightly closed and out of reach of children.
- Always read and follow all label warnings and cautions.
- Do not purchase essential oils with rubber glass dropper tops. Essential oils are highly concentrated and will turn the rubber to a gum, thus ruining the oil.
- Make note of when the bottle of essential oil was opened and its shelf life.
- Many essential oils will remove the furniture's finish. Use care when handling open bottles.
- Keep essential oil vials and clear glass bottles in a box or another dark place for storing.
- Be selective of where you purchase your essential oils. The quality of essential oil varies widely from company to company. Additionally, some companies may falsely claim their oils are undiluted and pure when they are not.

ESSENTIAL OIL SAFETY

In general, essential oils are safe to use for in the kitchen and therapeutic purposes. Nonetheless, safety must be exercised due to their potency and high concentration. Please read and follow these guidelines to obtain the maximum effectiveness and benefits.

- Be careful to avoid getting essential oils in the eyes. If you do splash a drop or two of essential oil in the eyes, use a small amount of olive oil (or another carrier oil) to dilute the essential oil and absorb with a wash cloth. If serious, seek medical attention immediately.

- If a dangerous quantity of essential oil has been ingested immediately drink olive oil and induce vomiting. The olive oil will help in slowing down its absorption and dilute the essential oil. Do not drink water – this will speed up the absorption of the essential oil.

- Pay attention to safety guidelines – certain essential oils, such as cinnamon and clove bud, may cause skin irritation for those with sensitive skin. If you experience slight redness or itchiness, put olive oil (or any carrier oil) on the affected area and cover with a soft cloth. The olive oil acts as an absorbent fat and binds to the oil diluting its strength and allowing it to be immediately removed. Redness or irritation may last 20 minutes to an hour.

- If you are pregnant, lactating, suffer from epilepsy or high blood pressure, have cancer, liver damage, or another medical condition, use essential oils under the care and supervision of a qualified Aromatherapist or medical practitioner.

- If taking prescription drugs, check for interaction between medicine and essential oils (if any) to avoid interference with certain prescription medications.

Tip:
Make sure the essential oils you use in your cooking, are steam-distilled at low temperatures and pressure (not carbon dioxide, solvents, or alcohol) and completely free of adulterants. Organic is ideal.

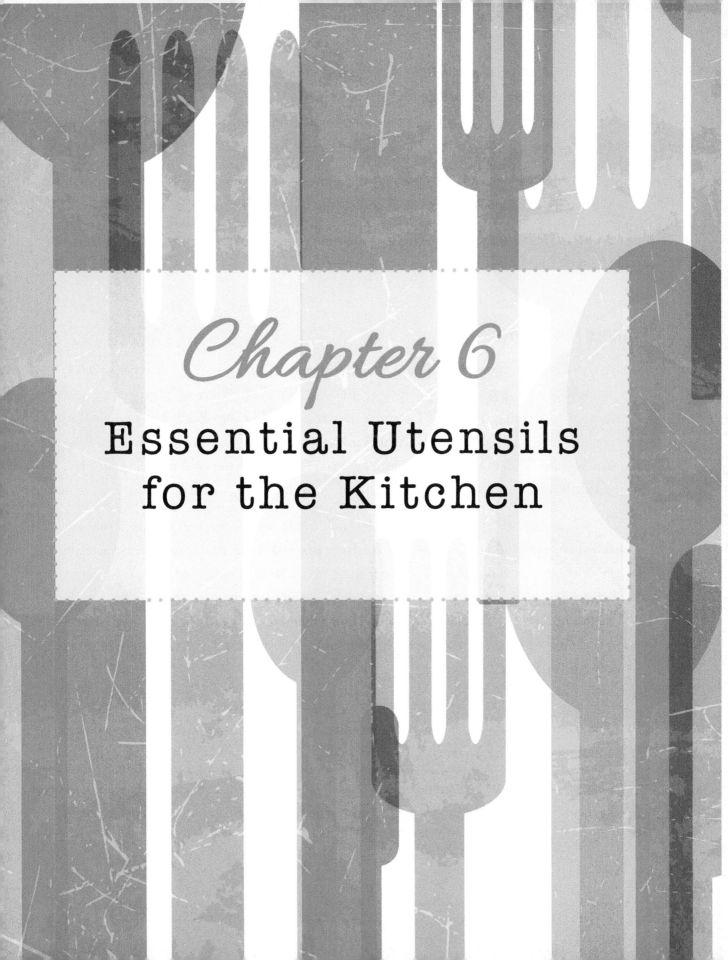

Chapter 6

Essential Utensils for the Kitchen

Different types of kitchen utensils and tools are used by both amateur and professional chefs. Procuring the most essential utensils for your kitchen will be necessary in preparing food. There are a multitude of cooking utensils and other tools available in the market today to choose from.

When cooking with essential oils use only glass, metal, or ceramic utensils and cookware for mixing and serving foods. Plastic may interact with or absorb the essential oil.

Are you lost in the myriad of different shapes and sizes of utensils and tools? Here is some of the basic equipment you will want to have in your kitchen to help ease your task of food preparation.

TOOLS FOR THE KITCHEN

Knives: Knives are an essential part of every kitchen. There are different types of knives available for cutting and chopping vegetables, carving, cutting bread, filleting and much more. If you own just one knife, you will want to make it a chef's knife. The midsize blade comes with a stocky, reinforced base that thins into a delicate tip that works as a multi-tool. You will also want to buy a knife-sharpener and get into the habit of sharpening your knife regularly. Dull knives make work for yourself by having to press harder.

Vegetable chopper: Chopping vegetables such as carrots, onions, and tomatoes can seem time-consuming and boring to many. However, nowadays vegetable choppers are available in different sizes and designs to suit individual needs. Both manual and electrical choppers are available that can be used to cut and dice vegetables in different shapes and sizes in a matter of minutes. They can also be used to cut different types of leaves and herbs. Hence, a vegetable chopper is a must for every kitchen. You will also need a vegetable peeler to peel various vegetables.

Cookware and utensils: Different types of utensils and cookware are required in a kitchen. These may include various types of pans and pots, non-stick cookware, cast iron cookware and stainless steel cookware.

Spoons and spatulas: Different types of spatulas and spoons form an essential part of every kitchen. Spoons are used to measure and distribute foods. Spatulas are used for mixing, blending, scraping, lifting, turning and raising foods. Spoons and spatulas are available in different sizes and materials.

Ladle: The ladle is a conventional kitchen utensil with a large long-handled spoon and a cup-shaped bowl that is used for serving soups and sauces.

Rolling pin: Another important part of every kitchen is the rolling pin. You will not be able to roll out and flatten your favorite pie crust without a rolling pin!

Mortar and Pestle: Mortar and pestle also are an essential requirement for your kitchen if you are fond of adding minced fresh herbs and spices to your meals. The mortar is a bowl, typically made of hard wood, ceramic or stone. The pestle is a heavy club-shaped object that is used for crushing and grinding. The substance to be ground is placed in the mortar and ground, crushed, or mixed with the pestle.

Electrical appliances: Different types of electrical appliances are also needed as part of a successful cooking experience. Food processors can cut and chop vegetables and fruits, make cookie dough, and grind spices and herbs. Juicers can be used to take the juice out of fruits and vegetables. Electrical egg beaters are used to make cake batter, beat eggs, and so forth. Toasters and grillers are used to toast and grill delicious sandwiches. Electric ovens are used to make pizzas, cakes, various types of meat and fish.

Bakeware: Apart from cooking utensils, different types of bakeware are also essential in a kitchen. You need oven-proof utensils for all your baking needs. These include cake pans, casserole dishes, baking trays and cookie sheets.

Kitchen scales: You may need to weigh different ingredients to prepare the perfect recipe. Hence, a small scale for weighing is also needed in your kitchen.

Oven or meat thermometer: To accurately cook meat you will need an oven or meat thermometer in your kitchen or pantry. This helps you know what the temperature is in the oven and when meat is completely cooked through.

Can opener: As a very small kitchen tool, a can opener can be easily forgotten. It is a handy device to open canned foods and is a definitely must have for your kitchen.

Fine-meshed strainer: A strainer is typically a steel bowl that has holes punched in it or is made of crossed wires that separates solid matter from a liquid. You will need a strainer to rinse vegetables or pasta. Look for a strainer or a colander that will hold very small pieces of food items.

Freestanding, four-sided box grater: You will need a grater to grate vegetables, cheese, and lemon and orange peels. You will want to ensure the grater you purchase makes a fine powder on one side, long skinny strands and short fat strands on the other two sides. To make cleanup easier, spritz your cheese grater with cooking spray before use.

Two cutting boards – one acrylic and one wood: You can use one side of your wooden cutting board to cut both dried and fresh fruits and the other side to cut herbs, garlic, vegetables and onion. This way your food will never taste of vegetables, especially garlic and onion. Use your acrylic cutting board to cut seafood, meat and poultry.

Pepper grinder: Proper seasoning is paramount. When a savory dish needs a little oomph, have a grinder on hand for adding fresh ground pepper.

Whisks: This is an important tool for beating or stirring a substance such as cream or eggs with a light, rapid movement.

Tools for handling essential oils: When using essential oils in your cooking, there are extra kitchen tools and utensils you will need. These include a small measuring spoon or glass dropper for measuring the exact drops of oil. In addition, you will need wooden toothpicks to add very minute quantities of essential oil to your dishes. You will want to store your essential oils in dark colored glass bottles in a dark, cool place.

Think about every stage of cooking from storage, cutting, cooking and presenting and you will get an idea of the utensils and tools that you will need in your kitchen. Cookware is available both online and at local department stores at readily affordable prices. Having what you need on hand will make your task much more enjoyable!

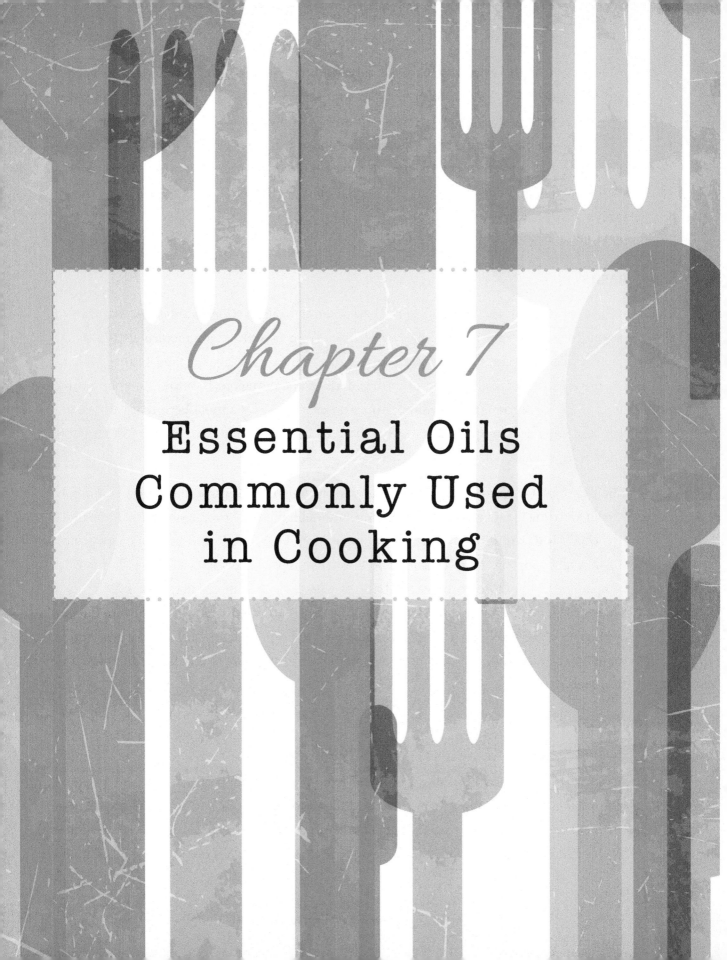

Chapter 7

Essential Oils Commonly Used in Cooking

What would pesto be without basil, or salsa without cilantro? You won't want to neglect adding a pinch of dried and fresh herbs to your favorite dishes, but essential oils can pull a recipe together by infusing the dish with unparalleled aroma and flavor. For example, Cooking Light's website suggest using basil's faint licorice flavor to brighten lemon sorbet, or rosemary's piney zing to complement chicken-zucchini skewers. Sometimes, when the effect you seek is subtle, refined, and delicate, a hint of essential oil is enough with just a swirl; other times, it takes a drop or two.

BASIL

Almost as popular as the dried herb, basil essential oil, or *Ocimum basilicum*, has gained prominence in recipes all over the world in cooking as well as for medicinal use. Basil's popularity in Europe, Central Asia, India and Southeast Asia has a long history with its extensive use for culinary purposes in the Mediterranean region. Basil oil is a good source of vitamin A, magnesium, potassium, iron, and calcium. This annual herb that can reach a height of three feet has pale pink to white flowers and big, rich herbaceous, almost balsamic woodsy scent.

The beautifully fragrant basil plant is abundant in Italian cookery, perhaps most commonly known for being the main ingredient in pesto. Although there are over 50 varieties of the herb, sweet basil is the most popular type for culinary use. Thai basil is also used in curry pastes, stir-fries and soups in Asian cuisine. The distinctive anise flavor of basil makes it a perfect companion to tomatoes, forming the basis of numerous Italian classics – such as Insalata Caprese. When used in cookery, basil is generally added towards the end, as its flavor is quickly destroyed. Alternatively, the raw leaves can be used to liven up salads and sandwiches. Add to soups and other savory dishes. A drop of basil oil is a simple way to add flavor and aroma to your food.

BAY LEAF

A jar of dried bay leaves is always a useful store-cupboard ingredient. Bay Leaf essential oil, or *Laurus nobilis*, can also be used to add flavor to pâté, stock and soups, particularly in Mediterranean and French cuisine. The most common type of bay leaf used in cookery is the bay laurel, which only develops its full flavor once dried. The leaves are usually cooked in the dish to impart flavor and then removed before eating. Contrary to popular belief, bay leaves are not toxic to consume but may be unpleasant to swallow due to their scratchy texture. For this reason, you may find it more convenient to use a drop or two of bay essential oil – thereby avoiding the need to fish out any unwanted leaves before serving.

BLACK PEPPER

Sourced from the dried berries of the *Piper nigrum* plant, black pepper is a key ingredient in any kitchen. Few restaurant tables are complete without their token salt and pepper shakers, making it one of the most popular seasonings in the world. For thousands of years, black pepper has been highly prized, even used as a currency and sacred offering by the ancient Greeks. The warm, spicy undertone of black pepper enhances the flavor of our food, while also improving digestion by preventing the formation of intestinal gas. It has also been proven to help break down fat cells, which may help with weight loss. Black pepper essential oil can be added to dips, sauces, and soups.

CELERY SEED

Celery is a common vegetable that is grown worldwide, not only for its crisp leaf stalks but also for its 'seeds,' which are actually tiny fruit. These celery seeds may be used as a spice to add flavoring to food, or ground with salt to create celery salt – a key ingredient in the classic Bloody Mary cocktail. Celery seeds are linked with health benefits such as lowering blood pressure and relieving pain. Celery features heavily in Creole and Cajun cuisine and serves as a key ingredient in the French mirepoix flavor base, which is at the heart of a variety of dishes. Celery seed essential oil, also known by its botanical name as *Apium graveolens*, can also be effective at detoxifying the liver and gallbladder.

CILANTRO

Love it or hate it, cilantro (also known as coriander) is abundant in many recipes, particularly in Mexican cuisine. Similar in appearance to flat-leaf parsley, cilantro is extremely versatile and beautifully enhances vegetables, meats, soups, curries and salads. Its distinctive pungency is an acquired taste that may divide your dinner guests! Cilantro is widely used across the world and is a key ingredient in many popular dishes such as guacamole and Indian dhal. Cultivated for thousands of years, its seeds are used as a spice, while its leaves are used as an herb. Cilantro is used in holistic medicine to aid digestion, and its essential oil, known in the botanical world as *Coriandrum satium*, has been shown to have antimicrobial properties.

CINNAMON

The wonderfully warm, spicy flavor of cinnamon is a baker's favorite and used in many sweet cakes, breads and pastries. Its evocative fragrance is associated with winter and Christmas time, often paired with ginger, vanilla or orange for a delicious warming synergy of aromas. Sourced from the bark of the cinnamon tree, the spice was treasured by the ancient Egyptians who considered it to be more precious than gold. As well as adding a unique flavor to food, cinnamon's antimicrobial properties make it an excellent food preservative, as well as helping to regulate blood sugar levels. You will find several different species to choose from – *Cinnamomum zeylanicum* and *Cinnamomum cassia blume*, are two favorites. Its versatility means you can have fun experimenting – try adding a drop of cinnamon essential oil to your morning coffee for an unusual twist. It can also be added to chocolate recipes for a luxurious treat!

CLOVE

Known for their sweet, aromatic warmth, cloves make an excellent addition to winter favorites such as gingerbread, mulled wine and pumpkin pie. They are a popular ingredient in Asian and Middle Eastern cookery, adding spice to meats, curries and bean soups. The sweet fragrance of cloves led to their use as breath fresheners in ancient China, where it was common for them to be chewed by courtiers. Clove essential oil, or *Syzygium aromaticum*, can be used to spice up candies, waffles and syrups. As a powerful antioxidant, cloves bring an array of health benefits that include aiding digestion, fighting bacteria and alleviating toothache.

CUMIN

The aromatic flavor of cumin is used to flavor curries in traditional Indian cuisine, as well as spicy Mexican and North African dishes. Cumin is often mistaken for caraway, as their names are extremely similar in many languages. It has been used since biblical times to aid digestion and headaches. The warming aroma of cumin oil, or *Cuminum cyminum*, is also beneficial for the nervous system, making it a wonderful ingredient in the kitchen. Cumin blends well with other spices, with a versatility that lends itself to so many dishes from soups to gravy – remember to use sparingly, as a little goes a long way.

DANDELION

The humble dandelion is far more than just a garden weed – its flowers and leaves are surprisingly nutritious and may be used in a variety of culinary and medicinal ways. Young dandelion leaves, known as 'greens,' have a mustard-like flavor which tastes great in salads. Older leaves can be cooked into soups or stews, providing a rich source of vitamins, iron, and calcium. In the 19th century, dandelion roots were roasted and ground into a powder that was used as a cheaper substitute for coffee. Its flowers may be used to make wine, jam, or medicinal honey, which is popular in Poland.

DILL

A common ingredient in European cuisine, the distinctive fresh flavor of dill lends itself to a range of foods including seafood, cream cheese, pickles and soups. The herb is most commonly known for its role in the Scandinavian dish gravlax, which combines the classic flavors of dill and salmon. As well as adding flavor, the carminative properties of dill essential oil, or *Anethum graveolens*, can ease digestion and relieve gas. In Poland, dill is one of the most popular kitchen herbs, where it is used to add flavor to dressings, soups and drinks. Dill is also widely used across Asia – particularly in India, where it is traditionally fed to new mothers following childbirth.

FENNEL

This deeply aromatic vegetable is characterized by its anise-like flavor that stems from anethole, a compound also found in star anise. In the culinary world, fennel makes a wonderful addition to salads, risottos and omelets. Its bulb, leaves and seeds are all useful flavoring ingredients. Fennel seed is widely used throughout Indian and Middle Eastern cookery, and is one of the essential components of Chinese five spice powder. Sugar-coated fennel seeds are a popular post-meal breath freshener in India and Pakistan. The carminative properties of fennel make it an excellent digestive aid, whether drank as a tea or eaten raw. Fennel essential oil, or *Foeniculum vulgare*, brings a spicy yet sweet taste that works well in bread recipes.

GARLIC

As the key ingredient for thousands of dishes, it is difficult to imagine a kitchen without garlic. From India to Italy, garlic plays a vital culinary role across the globe. It is a member of the Allium family and has been cultivated for more than 5,000 years. Today, garlic is as popular an ingredient as ever, bringing a unique aroma and flavor that is instantly recognizable. As well as enriching the taste of our food, garlic is also packed with health-giving properties, particularly when eaten raw. Most dishes can be enhanced with a touch of garlic, making it a must-have ingredient for any serious cook. Garlic essential oil, or *Allium sativum*, is a very powerful oil. Extreme care must be exercised when using.

GINGER

One of the most popular spices in the world, ginger has been prized for its medicinal and culinary benefits for thousands of years. The rich, spicy warmth of ginger works well in stir-frys and vegetable dishes, as well as sweet cakes and cookies. Ginger essential oil or, *Zingiber officinale*, is used in Ayurvedic cookery to improve the digestion of a meal, and helps to alleviate gastrointestinal problems. It is well known for its ability to reduce nausea and vomiting, particularly in pregnancy. In cookery, ginger particularly complements chocolate and citrus fruits, such as lemon, lime and orange. It is also fantastic for adding zing to fruit juices and smoothies. Because of ginger's versatility, it can be added to sweet and savory foods. For a savory taste, add to soups and stir-fries for an authentic Asian taste. For a sweet taste, add to chocolate sauces, biscuits and jams.

GRAPEFRUIT

An ancestor of the sweet orange, grapefruit has a sharp citrus flavor that is popular in salads and seafood recipes. A drop of grapefruit essential oil, or *Citrus racemosa*, can be added to fruit juices or cocktails for a tangy citrus twist, or mixed with olive oil to make a delicious salad dressing. Its refreshing flavor also works well in jams and palate-cleansing sorbets. Grapefruit can add an extra dimension to sweet dishes, coleslaw or beetroot salad – you can always mix with sweeter ingredients, such as orange, to balance out the flavors. Grapefruit essential oil can be added to water to help control appetite.

JUNIPER BERRY

The only spice to be sourced from a conifer, juniper berry is most famously known for providing the flavor of gin. The pinene content of juniper berry is responsible for its fresh, citrus-like aroma which has a great range of therapeutic benefits. It was used as a cheaper substitute for black pepper by the Romans and today is a popular ingredient in Northern European and Scandinavian cuisine, where it is commonly used to add flavoring to meat and game dishes. Some popular juniper berry recipes include meat terrine, game pie and duck confit. Try using juniper berry essential oil, also called *Juniperus communis* to add an unique twist to cocktails and desserts, such as mousses and jellies.

LAVENDER

Traditionally associated with fragrant massage oils and soaps, lavender should not be overlooked in the culinary world. Using lavender in the kitchen is a practice that dates back to the Middle Ages. Its essential oil can enhance savory dishes such as stews and sauces and is a good substitute for rosemary in bread recipes. When combined with oil and lemon juice, lavender creates an excellent marinade for pork or lamb. Lavender also blends very well with chocolate and makes for delightful syrups, cookies, ice creams and sorbets. Its colorful flowers add a beautiful garnish to salads or cocktails, with a soothing aroma that most people find deeply relaxing. You will discover a variety of lavender essential oils available on the market, *Lavandula angustifolia*, being one of the most popular.

LEMON

The refreshing flavor of lemon complements so many flavors in the kitchen, adding zest to both savory and sweet dishes from all over the world. Lemon essential oil, or *Citrus limon*, benefits from a far longer shelf-life than fresh juice, so any time a recipe calls for lemon flavor you can simply add one drop of oil. Its distinctive citrus scent not only tastes delicious but also uplifts the senses. The sharp flavor of lemon works particularly well with chicken and fish, as well as sweet dishes such as mousses, tarts and sorbets. For beginners, an easy way to start experimenting is by mixing one drop with olive oil to make a classic salad dressing. Lemon can be added to cakes, juices and teas.

LIME

Another member of the citrus family, lime makes a great substitution for its more popular cousin, the lemon. With a sweeter flavor, lime works particularly well in dessert and drink recipes. Adding just one drop of lime essential oil, or *Citrus aurantifolia*, can liven up the plainest glass of water, making it a useful store-cupboard ingredient. Make fruit salads and juices more exciting by adding a dash of lime, or add to stir-fries for an exotic twist. Try the classic combination of lime and ginger for a delicious cheesecake, or blend with a drop of mint for concocting a homemade mojito.

MANDARIN

A mandarin is a small citrus fruit, belonging to the same orange family as tangerines and satsumas. Usually eaten raw, mandarins can be enjoyed as a healthy snack or used in salads and desserts. Their taste is similar to orange, but usually sweeter and juicier. Chinese medicine uses the dried peel of mandarin as a remedy for digestive disorders. The fruits are traditionally exchanged at Christmas time, making it a popular ingredient during this season. Mandarin essential oil, or *Citrus reticulata*, can be used to add a delightful lemon-orange scent to drinks and desserts, such as fruit salads, jellies and mousses.

MARJORAM

It is believed that the ancient Greek goddess Aphrodite grew marjoram, which gave rise to its association with love potion recipes. These days, marjoram is a well-known herb used to flavor sauces, soups, stews and salad dressings. Commonly confused with its close relative oregano, marjoram adds a sweeter, milder flavor that is particularly suited to meat dishes. Burgers and bolognaise sauces can be livened up with a drop of marjoram essential oil, or *Origanum marjorana*, which replaces approximately 1 teaspoon of the dried herb. Marjoram tea is infused from its leaves and flowers, and traditionally used to treat digestive disorders.

NUTMEG

Sourced from the same tree as mace, nutmeg is an egg-shaped seed that is usually grated or used in powdered form in cookery. It is used in both sweet and savory recipes across the world, from Indian garam masala to Scottish haggis and the classic French potato dish gratin dauphinois. Also used in drinks, it is a key ingredient of eggnog and Caribbean rum cocktails. Although safe to consume in low doses, nutmeg contains myristicin – a psychoactive substance that, when consumed in large amounts, can be fatal. Fortunately, only a tiny amount of nutmeg oil, or *Myristica fragrans*, is required to impart a wonderful flavor.

ONION

Arguably one of the most fundamental ingredients in any kitchen, onions have been cultivated for around 7,000 years, for both medicinal and culinary use. The ancient Egyptians used onions as currency and buried them in the tombs of kings. Featuring in almost every global cuisine, they are prized for their versatile flavor and can be enjoyed in numerous ways, whether roasted, fried, stewed or eaten raw. As part of the Allium family, onions are rich in sulfur compounds that are responsible for that eye-watering, characteristic pungency. Rich in flavonoids, onions are packed with nutrients and deserve to be part of our daily diet. Onion essential oil, or *Allium cepa*, can be extremely strong and should always be used with extreme caution.

ORANGE

The sunny flavor of orange brings a sweet, fruity taste that has universal appeal. Bursting with vitamin C and other important nutrients, the delicious taste of orange can be enjoyed any time of day. A drop or two of orange essential oil, or *Citrus sinensis*, can be used as a substitute for the fresh ingredient. Classically paired with duck, orange also complements many fish and vegetable dishes, bringing a sweet sharpness that enhances the flavor of its accompanying ingredients. With such versatility, the opportunities for creativity in the kitchen are endless –

try adding a drop to cookie dough, ice cream or candies. For a jaffa taste, try adding orange essential oil to anything chocolate!

OREGANO

The classic pizza seasoning oregano is a staple of Italian and Greek cuisine. As a versatile herb, it can be used in a range of dishes from salads to sauces. It may be substituted for its close relative marjoram and brings a warm, slightly bitter flavor that complements roasted meat, fish and vegetables. Chopped oregano makes for a truly authentic Greek salad and can also be used to create wonderfully aromatic salad dressings. When cooking with oregano essential oil, or *Origanum compactum*, it is best added just at the end of cooking to maintain its flavor and aroma.

PARSLEY

The versatility of parsley makes it a must-have for any kitchen. Its mild, fresh flavor blends well with almost any dish, making it possibly the most ubiquitous herb in European and American cuisine. Curly parsley is often used as a garnish on salads, soups and stews, whereas the hardier flat parsley is more suited as a cooking ingredient. As well as adding a burst of color and flavor, parsley is also packed with vitamins and minerals, making it a super-healthy addition to any meal. Although safe in moderate amounts, excessive consumption of parsley should be avoided in pregnancy due to its potential labor-inducing effects. Parsley Seed Essential Oil, or *Petroselinum Sativum* does not smell at all like the culinary herb; it has a sweet, warm spicy scent that is herbaceous.

PEPPERMINT

The fresh taste of mint is a delightful addition to so many recipes, including desserts and drinks. Traditionally paired with lamb, mint also blends well with peas, carrots and other vegetables. Its leaves can be infused and drank as a refreshing tea, or crushed into cocktails, such as the traditional mint julep. Peppermint can also be added to anything chocolate to give it that choco-mint flavor and is great when combined with fresh lemon, too. The high menthol content of peppermint essential oil is responsible for its fresh, uplifting scent, which can be useful for treating nausea. Consuming fresh peppermint or using the essential oil such as *Mentha piperita* is also believed to aid digestive complaints, such as irritable bowel syndrome. Peppermint is identified by its rounded leaves, which are darker than the bright green leaves of its relative spearmint.

PETITGRAIN

Extracted from the leaves and twigs of the bitter orange tree, petitgrain, or *Citrus auratium*, has a similar fragrance to neroli and orange essential oil. Its fresh, uplifting scent can be used to add zest to drinks, desserts or sweet-and-sour recipes – a couple of drops is all it takes to transform the taste and aroma of a dish. Petitgrain works well with Thai flavors, so try adding it to stir-fries or salads. As a top note, petitgrain evaporates quickly, so remember to add it towards the end of cooking to preserve its flavor.

ROSE

Who can resist the alluring scent of rose, one of the most expensive and exquisite essential oils in the world? Rose is most famously used to make traditional Turkish delight, bringing a delicate yet distinctive flavor that has been enjoyed for hundreds of years. However, it can also be used to add a touch of luxury to syrups and desserts, or enjoyed as a refreshing tea. The gentle flavor works particularly well with ice cream, cupcakes and buttercream frosting. Due to its high cost, rose is often adulterated, so always look for pure, quality rose oil such as *Rosa damascena* when using in cookery.

ROSEMARY

Native to the Mediterranean, rosemary is an aromatic herb with distinctive needle-shaped leaves. Classically paired with roast lamb, it also blends well with Italian dishes such as focaccia bread and tomato-based sauces. With such a strong flavor, only a small amount is required – too much and the effect can be overpowering. Rosemary was cherished by the ancient Greeks for boosting the memory, and since then it has continued to be a popular herb that is commonly found in European cuisine. *Rosmarinus officinalis*, is considered a top note with a strong woody and herbal aroma and taste.

SAFFRON

Known as the 'king of spices,' saffron is the most expensive spice in the world. It is sourced from the saffron crocus flower or *Crocus sativa* and has been used in cookery, medicine and perfumery for over 3,000 years. The bright yellow color of saffron brings life to dishes such as the traditional Spanish paella. It is also a key ingredient in other classic recipes such as bouillabaisse and risotto alla Milanese. In Asia, it is mixed with milk and given to sick children to boost the immune system. When cooking with saffron, remember to use it sparingly, as over-consumption can cause nausea. Due to its high price tag, saffron is often adulterated, so always ensure you use pure, quality oil for culinary use.

SAGE

Originating from the Mediterranean region, sage is considered to be one of the main culinary herbs. With a flavor similar to lemon, mint and eucalyptus, it blends well with meat dishes – particularly turkey, pork, sausages and veal. Rosemary and thyme are good substitutes if sage is unavailable. One of the most well known culinary uses of the herb is for sage and onion stuffing, a classic combination that is the perfect addition to roast turkey at Thanksgiving or Christmas. Sage is not commonly used in French cookery, but is popular in British and Italian cuisine. Add to sauces, burger mixes and soups for a taste sensation. Sage essential oil, or *Salvia officinalis*, can be added to any existing savory recipe that calls for herbs and is especially delicious when essential oils and herbs are used together to enhance the flavor of the meal.

SPEARMINT

As a member of the mint family, spearmint, or *Mentha spicata*, has a cool, fresh flavor and aroma that serves as a fantastic flavoring for ice cream, confectionery and tea. Contrary to popular belief, an authentic mojito cocktail contains spearmint rather than peppermint leaves – although both work well. As with other varieties of mint, spearmint particularly complements lamb dishes and is very popular in Greek cuisine, where it is often used with cheese, tomatoes, rice and salads. Spearmint's leaves are bright green with a fuzzy appearance, easily distinguishable from its close relative peppermint. Its carminative properties make it useful in aiding digestion by preventing the formation of intestinal gas.

SAVORY

A reputed aphrodisiac, savory was used in cookery during the Middle Ages, when it was thought to be an effective treatment for gout, stomach complaints, toothache and ulcers. The high phenol content of its essential oil means it is strongly antiseptic, but should always be used sparingly. Its flavor is similar to thyme, although more punchy and bitter. Summer savory, or *Satureja hortensis*, is considered to be more suited to cookery than its winter equivalent. Great with grilled meats and fish, or drank as a refreshing herbal tea, savory is one of the more unusual ingredients to experiment with in your kitchen.

TANGERINE

Closely related to mandarin, tangerine, or *Citrus nobilis*, a citrus fruit with a sweeter flavor than the classic orange. Its name derives from its origins in Tangier, a city in Morocco. With a calming aroma and a sweet, tangy taste, tangerine makes a lovely addition to fruit salads or fruity curry dishes. Its essential oil is rich in antioxidants and can be added to food as a substitute for fresh orange juice or extract. Its fresh, uplifting scent will add zest to all types of casseroles, stir-fries and soups. As with other top notes, tangerine oil will evaporate quickly, so always add just before the food is served.

TARRAGON

Fresh tarragon has a distinctively bittersweet, licorice-like flavor, which blends well with fish, chicken and omelets. Popular in French cookery, tarragon is one of the key ingredients in the classic béarnaise sauce. Like most herbs, several varieties exist; however, for culinary use French tarragon, or *Artemisia dracunculus*, is considered to be the best. The fresh herb or oil can be used to flavor vinegars and butters, or eaten raw in salads, contrasting nicely with other fresh herbs such as parsley and chives. A good substitute is fennel, which has a similar anise flavor.

THYME

As one of the most commonly used herbs in the kitchen, thyme blends beautifully with other herbs such as parsley, sage and rosemary. French thyme is the most popular variety, also known as 'common' or 'garden' thyme, which has a wide range of culinary and medicinal uses. The herb is hugely popular in Cajun and Creole cooking and is a key ingredient in any chef's classic bouquet garni. As well as bringing an aromatic, earthy tone to roasted meats, thyme essential oil can also add a twist to omelets or scrambled eggs, as well as stews, stuffings and marinades. Thyme essential oil is used to flavor meats, soups and stews. It is often used as a primary flavor with lamb, tomatoes, and eggs. White Thyme is more commonly derived from the *Thymus zygis* species, while Red Thyme essential oil comes from *Thymus vulgaris* species. Dilution is necessary as this oil can possibly irritate the mucous membranes. For sore throat teas, dilute one drop in two teaspoons of honey or in 8 ounces of beverage.

TURMERIC

A member of the ginger family, turmeric is a popular spice that is known for its vivid yellow coloring, which enhances the taste and appearance of dishes across South Asia. For thousands of years, turmeric has been used in Ayurvedic medicine as a remedy to treat a range of illnesses, including digestive disorders. It is one of the key ingredients in most standard curry powders, bringing a slightly bitter, peppery taste that complements most meat, fish and vegetable dishes. Turmeric is mainly used in savory recipes, although it can be used as flavoring in some Asian cakes and desserts. Turmeic essential oil comes from the species, *Curcuma longa* and is viewed as a strong relaxant.

VANILLA

The delicious, sensual scent of vanilla has universal appeal, with a sweetness that brings life to so many recipes in the kitchen. It is the second most expensive spice in the world after saffron, as the process of cultivating vanilla pods is so labor-intensive. Popular with children and adults alike, vanilla can be added to all sorts of recipes from ice cream to cakes, cookies and custard. Its essential oil is much stronger than regular vanilla extract, so use with care – one drop is often all you need. Vanilla-flavored syrups are a great way to enjoy its delicious flavor in coffees and milkshakes. Vanilla comes from the *Vanilla planifolia* species and is known as one of the most popular aromas, with a comforting and relaxing scent.

ESSENTIAL OILS FLAVOR GROUPS

Minty Flavors: Peppermint, Spearmint

Floral Flavors: Geranium, Rose, Lavender

Herbal Flavors: Oregano, Basil, Dill, Rosemary, Sage, Tarragon

Tangy Flavors: Lemon, Orange, Lime, Tangerine, Petitgrain, Grapefruit, Mandarin

Spicy Flavors: Cinnamon, Clove Bud, Nutmeg, Ginger, Black Pepper, Cardamom, Cumin

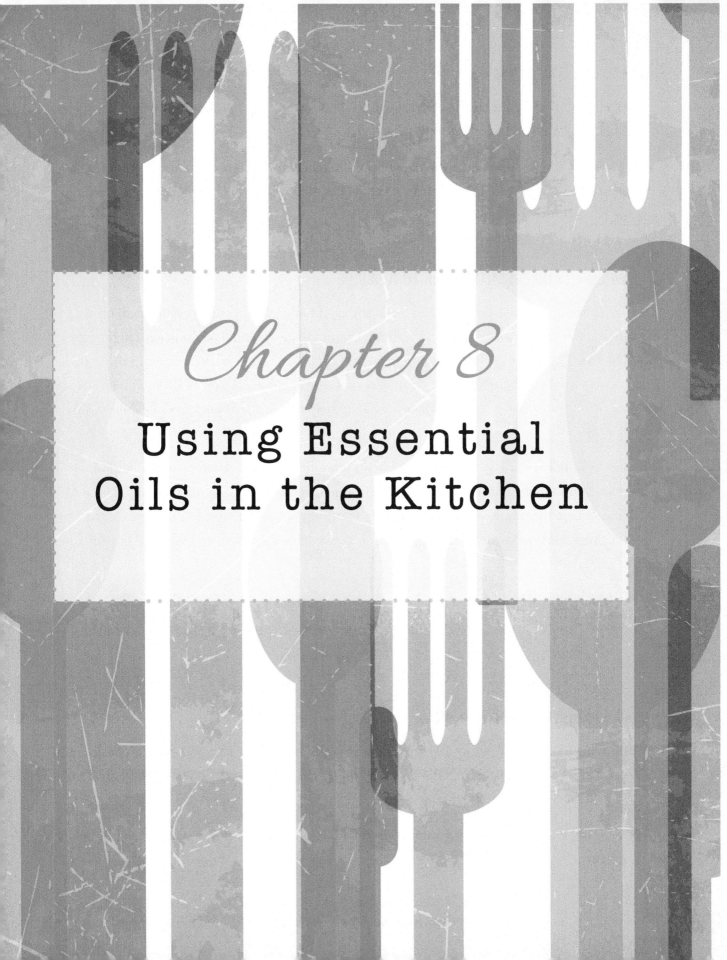

Chapter 8
Using Essential Oils in the Kitchen

HOW MUCH DO I USE?

Always start off by adding one drop at a time. This is when the "less is more" principle applies. You can always add another drop if needed.

Adding the right amount can make all the difference in the flavor of your dish. For recipes that serve 6-10 people, 1-2 drops of essential oil is plenty. You can add more or less depending upon your taste and preference.

WHEN TO ADD ESSENTIAL OILS TO A RECIPE

When using essential oils in a recipe, add the essential oil right before serving so to maximize their flavor impact and so the heat does not evaporate the essential oil's nutrients in the steam. Heartier essential oils like thyme, oregano and rosemary can be added earlier in the cooking process to allow their flavors to completely infuse your dish. If you find the added oils are too strong, you may want to simmer a while to help tone it down and produce a more subtle bouquet.

Just as it makes sense to "season" foods with salt and pepper at different stages of cooking, it makes sense to add essential oils at different times to take advantage of the unique qualities. A little experimentation and you'll quickly learn how to get the results you desire. For salad dressings, marinades, desserts and other non-cooked items, you can add essential oils anytime.

 Tip:
For best results, add essential oils during the final steps of the cooking process, unless the recipe directs otherwise.

ESSENTIAL OILS AND HIGH HEAT

Cooking temperatures above 104 degrees F/40 degrees C may destroy some of the constituents in essential oils causing them to lose some of their healing benefits. You will still add great taste to your casserole or entrée, though.

One way to prevent this is to add the essential oil at the end of the cooking time, just before serving.

HOW TO ADD ESSENTIAL OILS TO A RECIPE

Adding too many drops of essential oil can ruin your dish! Especially when you are adding thin oils that comes out of the bottle fast. To prevent this from happening, add a couple of tablespoons of your soup or casserole into a small cup. Add one or two drops of essential oil to the cup and stir to mix well. Pour the mixture back in with the original dish and voila! If by chance you do add too many drops of essential oil into small cup, you will have only lost a few tablespoons of dinner, not the entire meal.

Another method to use when adding essential oil to your dish is to drop the oil onto a spoon and then stir in, instead of directly into the pan.

 Tip:
Always mix essential oils into another liquid in a separate bowl. This way, when they are added into the dish they will be evenly distributed in your dish.

DILUTION OF ESSENTIAL OILS

As a general rule, always dilute one drop of essential oil in one teaspoon of honey, vegetable oil, or sauce before adding to a dish or entrée. When adding an essential oil to a beverage, use two to four ounces of liquid for dilution.

For stronger oils such as basil, marjoram, oregano, or thyme or for a more subtle flavor, you will want to use the "toothpick method" when adding essential oils to your dish.

TOOTHPICK METHOD

When one drop is still too much, try dipping a wooden toothpick in the bottle of essential oil (remove the plastic reducer cap if necessary) then swirl it in the dish or sauce at the end of cooking or just before serving.

Tip:
Keep in mind, when flavoring your food with essential oil, two drops of essential oil is equivalent to a full two-ounce bottle of dried herbs.

ESSENTIAL OIL COOKING

- Only use 100% pure, preferably organic essential oils. Choose only oils that are included on the FDA's GRAS list.

- When adding an essential oil to a recipe, always mix in with a vegetable oil, honey, or another liquid, to help disperse the essential oil more evenly.

- Warm oils such as cinnamon, clove bud, thyme, and oregano can cause irritation if they come into direct contact with the skin or mucous membranes and should always be diluted when used. These oils, however, do not pose any problem when mixed evenly in with food.

- Oils such as thyme, oregano and wintergreen should never be used in quantities more than one drop.

- When using essential oils in a recipe, add the essential oil right before serving to maximize their flavor impact and so the heat does not evaporate essential oils in the steam.

- For recipes that serve 6-10 people, add 1-2 drops of essential oil and stir in after cooking or just before serving so the oil's nutrients will not be lost in evaporation.

- Always mix essential oils into another liquid in a separate bowl. This way they will be evenly distributed in your dish.

- For best results, add essential oils during the final steps of the cooking process, unless the recipe directs otherwise.

- Don't know how much to make? Allow 4-6 appetizers per guest if the meal quickly follows. When a meal is late, allow 6-8 pieces per guest. If no meal is planned, allow 8-10 appetizers per guest.

- For vinaigrette, the typical ratio is 3 parts vegetable oil to 1 part vinegar.

- Chill serving plates to keep salads crisp. Perk up soggy lettuce by spritzing it with a mixture of lemon essential oil and cold water.

- When serving soup as a main dish, count on 1/2 quart per person. When served as an appetizer or side dish, count on 1 quart serving six.

- Always chill juices before adding them to beverage recipes.
- When making fresh lemonade or orange juice, one lemon yields about 1/4 cup juice, while one orange yields about 1/3 cup juice.

CONVERSION GUIDELINES

CITRUS JUICE OR ZEST

When using an essential oil in place the zest of "one" whole lemon, orange, or tangerine, use 8 to 14 drops of its companion essential oil.

Zest of one whole fruit = 8-14 drops of its companion essential oil

DRIED SPICES

One tablespoon of dried herb/spice is equivalent to 1/2 to 1 drop of essential oil. When a recipe calls for less than a teaspoon of an herb or dried spice, use the toothpick method to add essential oil to your recipe or beverage.

One tablespoon of dried herb/spice = 1/2 to 1 drop of its companion essential oil

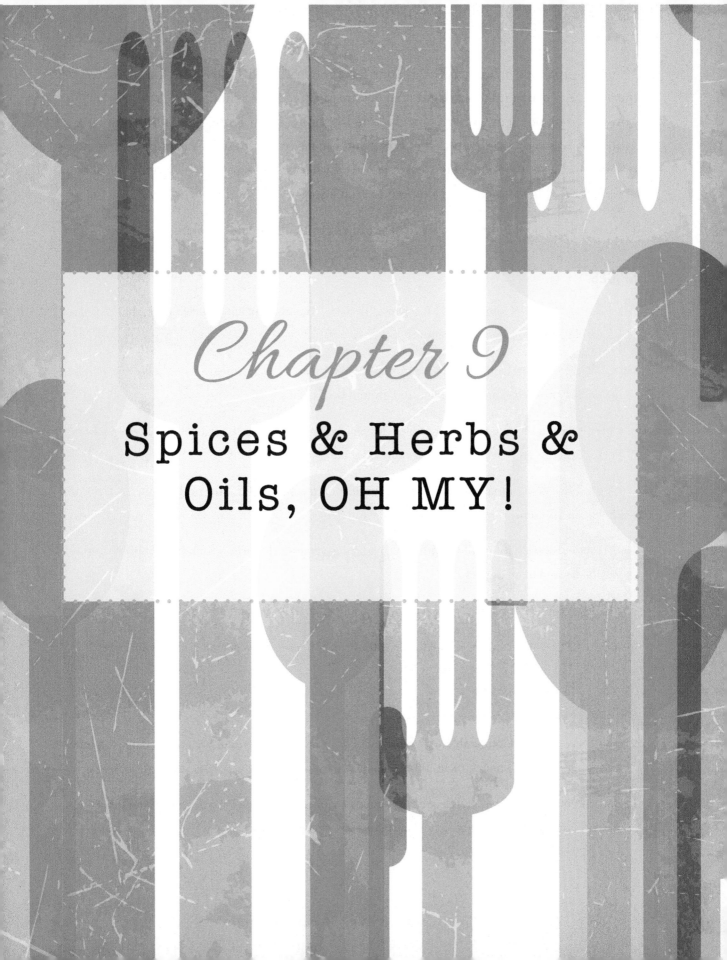

Chapter 9

Spices & Herbs & Oils, OH MY!

Using essential oils or fresh herbs in your favorite dish will definitely enhance its flavor or nutrition. Keep in mind though, essential oils are much more potent than fresh or dried herbs. You can combine them with fresh or dried herbs, or use them in place of a called-for spice. Only one or two drops are needed to create intense flavor and in some cases for hot essential oils, you will want to use the toothpick method. For herbs, 1/3 teaspoon of ground herbs or 1 teaspoon dried herbs is equal in strength to 1 tablespoon fresh herbs.

Here is a list of some of the ways you can add essential oils in your cooking:

SPICES

Allspice — Sweet. Compatible with fruits, desserts, breads, duckling, beef, pork, ham, yellow vegetables, tomato sauces and relishes.

Cinnamon — Sweet. Compatible with fruits, desserts, breads, tomato-meat sauces, yellow vegetables, beverages, pork, chicken, some beef and ground beef dishes.

Clove — Sweet and pungent. Compatible with pickled fruits, desserts, baked goods, beverages, lamb, pork, corned beef, tongue, yellow vegetables, tomato sauces and beets.

Ginger — Sweet. Compatible with fruits, squash, poultry, sauces for fish, pork, some beef dishes, cheese and desserts.

Nutmeg — Sweet. Compatible with fruits, eggnog, cheese, desserts, ground beef, poultry, most vegetables and many sauces.

Paprika — Mild. Compatible with beef, poultry, soups, salads, eggs and goulash.

Saffron — Pungent, aromatic. Compatible with meat, fish, poultry, vegetables, sauces and rice.

HERBS

Basil — Sweet, mild. Compatible with cheeses, pesto, vegetables, particularly green beans, tomatoes and tomato sauces, poultry, meat, rabbit, potato salads and sauces.

Bay — Sweet, mellow. Compatible with any foods requiring a bouquet garni, court bouillon, soups, stews, vegetables, pickling and other marinades and spaghetti sauce.

Chives – Mild, onionlike. Compatible with sauces, salad dressings, cream, mild fish, poultry and veal.

Dill – Mild. Compatible with fish, particularly salmon, pork, cottage cheese, potatoes, sauerkraut and other cabbage dishes, cauliflower, beans, pickles and sauce.

Marjoram – Sweet, mild. Compatible with meat, particularly lamb, poultry, stuffings, cheese, vegetables, tomato-based sauces, soups and rabbit.

Mint – Strong, aromatic. Compatible with meats, vegetables, fruits, beverages and salads.

Oregano – Spicy, pungent. Compatible with tomato dishes, fish, especially red snapper, vegetables used in Italian cuisine, stews, chili, beef and pork dishes.

Parsley – Mild. Compatible with court bouillon soups, stews, meat, poultry, fish, sauces, cheese, many vegetables and eggs.

Rosemary – Strong, acrid. Compatible with duckling, poultry, meat, fish, stuffings and some vegetables like spinach, mushrooms, carrots, tomatoes and beans.

Sage – Strong. Compatible with stuffings, pork, poultry, tomatoes, rice dishes and Brussel sprouts.

Tarragon – Mild. Compatible with fish, poultry, lamb, veal, salad dressings, vinegars, potato salads, and some vegetables like beans, mushrooms and spinach. Essential for Béarnaise sauce.

Thyme – Pungent, aromatic. Compatible with soups, stews, stuffings, rice dishes, Mediterranean vegetables, dishes with red wine and/or tomatoes, rabbit, veal, lamb, fish and poultry.

Adding flavor to your favorite entrée or dish is really simple with essential oils. Here's a few suggestions to help you get started:

Salad Dressings or Marinades: Lemon, lavender, rosemary, clove bud or peppermint in a vegetable oil. As a general rule of thumb, add 1 drop of essential oil to 1 teaspoon of vegetable oil.

Meats, Sauces, Rubs: Basil, marjoram, oregano, sage, or thyme. For brushed-on marinades, add 1 drop of essential oil to 1 tablespoon of vegetable oil. Strong meats are especially enhanced with essential oil.

Fruit Wash: Lemon, lime, tangerine, mandarin, petitgrain, or grapefruit essential oil.

Fish and Seafood: Black pepper, fennel, lavender, lemon, lime, orange, parsley, rosemary, sage, or thyme essential oil.

Poultry: Basil, dill, fennel, lemon, marjoram, melissa, orange, oregano, parsley, rosemary, sage, tarragon, or thyme essential oil.

Cakes, Frosting, Puddings, Pies: Lemon, clove bud, orange, tangerine, or peppermint essential oil.

Herbal Teas: Lavender, roman chamomile, orange, tangerine, lemon, peppermint, or melissa essential oil.

Cool Refreshing Drinks: Lemon, orange, tangerine, or peppermint. Add essential oil to a pitcher of water with slices of fruit added for color.

Flavored Honey: Cinnamon, clove bud, lavender, basil, roman chamomile, or lemon essential oil. Warm the honey until it becomes a thin liquid then add the essential oil and stir to blend.

Desserts: Cardamom, cinnamon, clove bud, grapefruit, lavender, lemon, lime, mandarin, nutmeg, orange, peppermint, spearmint, or tangerine essential oil.

Source: Evelyn Vincent, The Very Essence Blog
http://theveryessence.com/pdf/Cooking_with_Essential_Oils_Guidelines.pdf

HERB AND SPICE SUBSTITUTION CHARTS

While creating dinner one night you may suddenly realize you are out of a specified spice called for in a recipe or perhaps you just don't care for that particular spice. Use these charts to help you choose a suitable substitution that will work well with your recipe.

When you do substitute an essential oil for a spice or herb, you will quickly realize that the flavor will not be as originally intended in the recipe. Because of this, it is a good idea to begin with just a swirl of essential oil using the "toothpick method." If you intend on using a dried herb or spice instead, you will want to use only half the specified recipe amount and then adjust to your own personal tastes. Feel free to adjust the amount and add to any recipe that suites you and your family. Who knows? You may create a new family favorite!

Spice Substitutions

Allspice	Cinnamon, Cassia, Nutmeg, Mace, or Cloves
Aniseed	Fennel or Aniseed
Cardamom	Ginger
Chili Powder	Hot Pepper Sauce (bottled) plus Oregano and Cumin
Cinnamon	Nutmeg or Allspice (use only 1/4 of the amount)
Clove	Allspice, Cinnamon, or Nutmeg
Cumin	Chili powder
Ginger	Allspice, Cinnamon, Mace, or Nutmeg
Mace	Allspice, Cinnamon, Ginger, or Nutmeg
Mustard (dry)	Wasabi powder (1/4 to 1/2 as much since it is hotter), or Horseradish powder; 1 teaspoon dry mustard powder = 1 tablespoon prepared mustard
Nutmeg	Cinnamon, Ginger, or Mace
Saffron	Turmeric or Annato powder (for color)
Turmeric	Saffron (for color) plus Mustard powder, or Annato powder

Herb & Root Substitutions

Basil	Oregano or Thyme
Chervil	Tarragon or Parsley
Chives	Green Onions (scallions), Onion, or Leek
Cilantro	Parsley
Dill	Basil, Chervil, Parsley, or Tarragon
Fennel	Aniseed, Basil, Cumin, Garlic, Onion, Rosemary, or Thyme
Garlic	Black Pepper, Celery, Cumin, Fennel, Ginger, Horseradish, Onion, Scallions, or Leek
Italian Seasoning	Blend of any of these: Basil, Oregano, Rosemary, and Red Pepper (ground)
Marjoram	Basil, Thyme, or Savory
Mint	Basil, Marjoram, or Rosemary
Oregano	Thyme or Basil
Parsley	Chervil or Cilantro
Poultry Seasoning	Sage plus a blend of any of these: Thyme, Marjoram, Savory, Black Pepper, and Rosemary
Red Pepper Flakes (dried)	Hot Pepper Sauce (bottled) or Black Pepper
Rosemary	Thyme, Tarragon, or Savory
Sage	Poultry seasoning, Savory, Marjoram, or Rosemary
Savory	Thyme, Marjoram, or Sage

Herb & Root Substitutions	
Tarragon	Chervil, Fennel, or Aniseed
Thyme	Basil, Marjoram, Oregano, or Savory

EMERGENCY SUBSTITUTIONS

Although best results are achieved when using the ingredients called for in a recipe, emergency situations may arise where you are in a pinch and need to substitute an ingredient. Keep in mind, end results may vary.

Baking	
Ingredient	**Substitution**
1 teaspoon baking powder	1/4 teaspoon baking soda plus 1/2 teaspoon cream of tartar
1 package active dry yeast	1 tablespoon dry or 1 cake compressed yeast, crumpled
1 cup honey	1 1/4 cups sugar plus 1/4 cup liquid
1 cup cake flour	1 cup sifted all-purpose flour minus 2 tablespoons
1 cup oil	1/2 pound butter or margarine
1 cup brown sugar	1 cup granulated sugar

Dairy	
Ingredient	**Substitution**
1 cup whole milk	1/2 cup evaporated milk plus 1/2 cup water, or 1 cup reconstituted nonfat dry or skim milk plus 2 teaspoons butter or oil
1 cup buttermilk or sour milk	1 tablespoon cider vinegar or lemon juice plus enough milk to equal 1 cup and allowed to stand 5 minutes
1 cup dairy sour cream	1 cup plain yogurt or 1 cup evaporated milk plus 1 tablespoon vinegar, or 1 cup cottage cheese mixed in a blender with 2 tablespoons milk and 1 tablespoon lemon juice
1 cup half and half	7/8 cup milk plus 3 tablespoons margarine or butter, or 1 cup evaporated milk

Vegetables

Ingredient	Substitution
1 cup canned tomatoes	1 1/3 cups fresh-cut tomatoes, simmered 10 minutes
1 cup tomato sauce	8-ounce can stewed tomatoes, blended in a blender or 1 cup tomato puree seasoned or 3/4 cup tomato paste plus 1/4 cup water
1/2 pound fresh mushrooms	4-ounce can mushrooms
Legumes	Any dried beans can be used (except lentils)

Herbs and Spices

Ingredient	Substitution
1 tablespoon fresh herbs	1 teaspoon same herb, dried or 1/4 teaspoon ground or powdered
1 teaspoon dry mustard	2 teaspoons prepared mustard
1 teaspoon pumpkin pie spice	1/2 teaspoon dried cinnamon, 1/2 teaspoon ginger, 1/8 teaspoon ground allspice, 1/8 teaspoon nutmeg

Thickeners

Ingredient	Substitution
1 tablespoon cornstarch	2 tablespoons flour, or 1/3 tablespoon quick cooking tapioca
1 tablespoon flour	1/2 tablespoon cornstarch, or 2 teaspoons quick cooking tapioca, or two egg yolks
1 tablespoon tapioca	1 1/2 tablespoons all purpose flour

Chapter 10
Appetizers

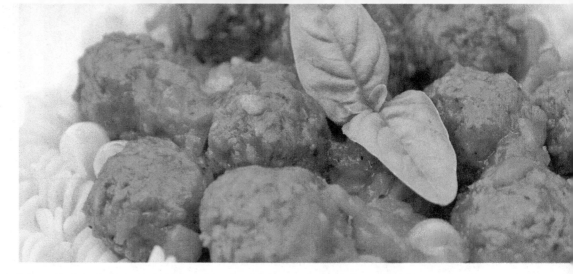

MEATBALLS WITH GARLIC, ONION AND LEMON OIL

Serves 4

Savory meatballs infused with lemon, garlic, and onion bring a mouthful of flavor to this appetizer. These can be served with the marinara sauce which takes very little time to make!

RECOMMENDED ESSENTIAL OILS:

3-5 drops of lemon oil

WHAT YOU WILL NEED:

1 lb. lean ground beef

2 cloves fresh garlic, minced

1 tsp. Italian seasoning

1/2 tsp. onion powder

1 lemon, zested (or 3 drops lemon essential oil)

1/4 - 1/2 cup Italian flavored breadcrumbs

2 eggs

Olive oil

Salt and pepper to taste

FOR THE MARINARA SAUCE:

28-ounce can whole tomatoes with juice

2 cloves fresh garlic, thinly sliced

1 shallot, chopped

1 tbsp. extra virgin olive oil

1/2 tsp. dried oregano

1 tsp. dried basil

1/2 tsp. salt

WHAT TO DO:

1. Set ground beef and eggs out on counter for 10-15 minutes so they aren't freezing cold (your hands will thank you later).

2. Pour olive oil into a large frying pan, covering the bottom with about 1/2 inch of oil. Preheat over low heat.

3. In a large bowl, add all of the meatball ingredients, minus the sauce and half of the breadcrumbs.

4. Add the essential oil into the bowl. Blend well.

5. Using your bare hands, mix all of the ingredients together. If the mixture is too moist, add more breadcrumbs until you can easily form meatballs.

6. Take an ice cream scoop and scoop up meat mixture. Then, roll in your hands to form a ball. Place them in the frying pan.

7. Once all the meatballs have been added to the pan, raise the heat to a medium. Cook until golden brown, approximately 3-5 minutes on each side.

8. Place cooked meatballs on a plate lined with a paper towel to drain excess fat.

9. Place tomatoes and their juice in a food processor fitted with the metal blade (or a blender) and process for 30-60 seconds for a chunky sauce. If you prefer a smoother sauce, process longer.

10. In a small saucepan, heat the olive oil over medium-high heat; add the garlic and shallots and sauté for about one minute. Add tomatoes, oregano, basil and salt. Simmer over low heat, stirring occasionally for about 10 minutes.

11. Pour marinara sauce into a shallow serving dish. Serve meatballs with toothpicks for dipping in marinara sauce.

CRAB CAKES WITH LEMON, BLACK PEPPER AND PARSLEY OIL

Serves 6–8

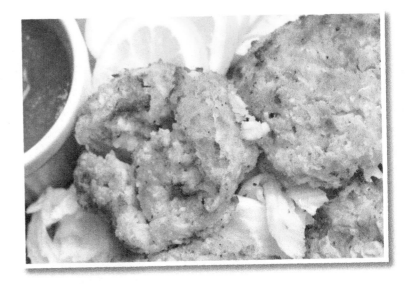

Lemon and parsley infused crab cakes bring just the right balance for the crispy texture of the breadcrumbs and tasty crab inside.

RECOMMENDED ESSENTIAL OILS:

1 drop of parsley oil
1 drop of lemon oil
1 drop of black pepper oil

WHAT YOU WILL NEED:

2/3 cup real mayonnaise
5 egg yokes
3 tbsp. fresh parsley, chopped (or 1 drop parsley essential oil)
2 tbsp. Worcestershire sauce
2 tsp. mustard
2 tsp. lemon juice (or 1 drop lemon essential oil)

2 tsp. black pepper (or 1 drop black pepper essential oil)
Salt to taste
1/4 tsp. blackening seasoning
1/2 tsp. crushed red pepper
2 1/2 - 3 cups seasoned breadcrumbs
2 lbs. fresh lump crabmeat
Canola oil

WHAT TO DO:

1. Preheat a skillet over medium heat with about 1/2 inch of canola oil. In a large bowl, combine the mayonnaise, mustard, Worcestershire sauce and seasonings.

2. Add chopped parsley (or essential oil), then stir in the fresh ground black pepper (or essential oil).

3. Next, squeeze lemon juice into the mixture (or essential oil) and stir.

4. Finally, add in crabmeat, egg yolks, and breadcrumbs, reserving 1/2 cup of breadcrumbs for later. Mix well.

5. Using an ice cream scoop, take some of the crabmeat mixture into your hand to form a crab cake. If the meat doesn't hold together, add remaining breadcrumbs.

6. Place crab cakes in the skillet to brown on each size, cooking 3-5 minutes. Once done, drain on a paper towel and serve hot.

STUFFED MUSHROOMS WITH PARSLEY AND ONION OIL

Serves 6

Mushrooms have a way of soaking up flavors, and with the onion, parsley and oregano in these baked with butter and Parmesan cheese, it is hard to just eat one.

RECOMMENDED ESSENTIAL OILS:

1 drop of onion oil
1 drop of parsley oil

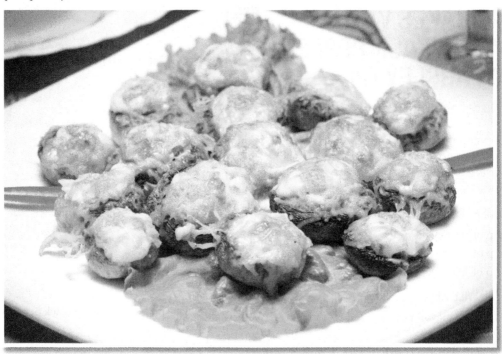

WHAT YOU WILL NEED:

1 small package fresh mushrooms (larger ones are best)

3 tbsp. butter

1/4 cup celery, diced

2 tbsp. onions, diced (or 1 drop onion essential oil)

1/2 cup seasoned breadcrumbs

1 tsp. Worcestershire sauce

Dash of salt

1 tsp. parsley flakes (or 1 drop parsley essential oil)

1 tsp. fresh oregano, chopped

1/4 cup freshly grated Parmesan cheese

WHAT TO DO:

1. Preheat oven to 350 degrees. While oven preheats, remove the stems from the mushroom caps and wash well. Chop stems and dice celery and onions.

2. In a medium skillet, melt the butter. Add diced onions (or essential oil) and parsley flakes (or essential oil), diced celery, onions and mushroom stems. Saute until they become soft. Once softened, remove from heat.

3. Add the breadcrumbs, Worcestershire sauce, salt and oregano. Mix well.

4. Place mushroom caps on a greased cookie sheet, cap down. Stuff each cap with the breadcrumb mixture. Top each mushroom with cheese. Bake 8-10 minutes until mushroom caps are soft.

7 LAYER DIP WITH ONION, CILANTRO AND GARLIC OIL

Serves 12

This dip has a little bit of everything, which when combined makes for the perfect dip. Infused with cilantro, garlic and onion this dip comes to life with flavor.

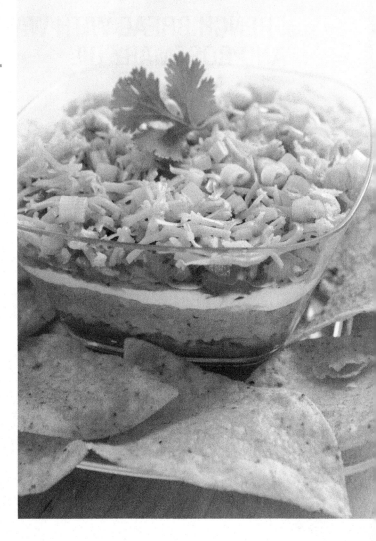

RECOMMENDED ESSENTIAL OILS:

1 drop of cilantro (or coriander) oil

1 drop of garlic oil

WHAT YOU WILL NEED:

1 can refried beans

1 heaping cup sour cream

1 heaping cup guacamole

1 heaping cup salsa

1 bunch green onions, chopped

1 cup cheddar cheese

1 small can black olives, sliced

1 cup fresh tomatoes, diced

1 tbsp. fresh cilantro (or 1 drop cilantro essential oil)

3 cloves garlic, minced (or 1 drop garlic essential oil)

1 package taco seasoning

WHAT TO DO:

1. In a bowl, add taco seasoning and sour cream. Mix well.

2. In another bowl, add salsa and cilantro (or essential oil). Stir well.

3. In another bowl, add chopped onions with the beans.

4. In another bowl, add minced garlic (or essential oil) with guacamole.

5. Once all the layers are ready, add each one into a clear glass bowl layering as follows: beans, sour cream, guacamole, sour cream, salsa, cheese and green onions. Refrigerate 1 hour before serving.

FRENCH BREAD WITH WARM GOAT CHEESE AND ROSEMARY OIL

Serves 8

This warm, creamy goat cheese spread sprinkled with fresh herbs is the perfect companion for slices of a baguette.

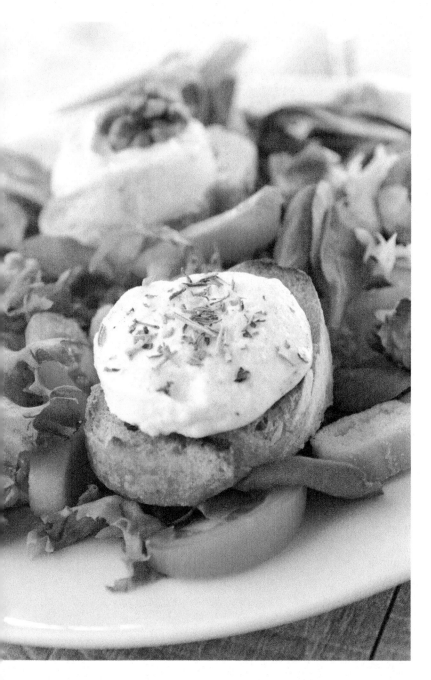

RECOMMENDED ESSENTIAL OILS:

1 drop of rosemary oil

WHAT YOU WILL NEED:

1 fresh French baguette, sliced

8 ounces soft fresh goat cheese

1/4 cup honey

1/2 tbsp. fresh rosemary, chopped (or 1 drop rosemary essential oil)

WHAT TO DO:

1. Preheat oven to 350 degrees. Take approximately 1 ounce of goat cheese and smooth it onto each slice of bread.

2. Lay each slice onto a baking sheet and bake approximately 7 minutes until the bread is lightly toasted and cheese is soft.

3. While the bread is baking, heat the honey with fresh rosemary (or essential oil) in a small sauce pan until hot.

4. Drizzle the bread with the honey mixture as soon as it comes out of the oven. Top with fresh chopped rosemary if you'd like and serve right away while warm.

STUFFED JALAPEÑO PEPPERS WITH SAGE OIL

Serves 12

This spicy, snappy blend is hard to resist. Infusing the cream cheese and freshly chopped sage adds another dimension to the flavor.

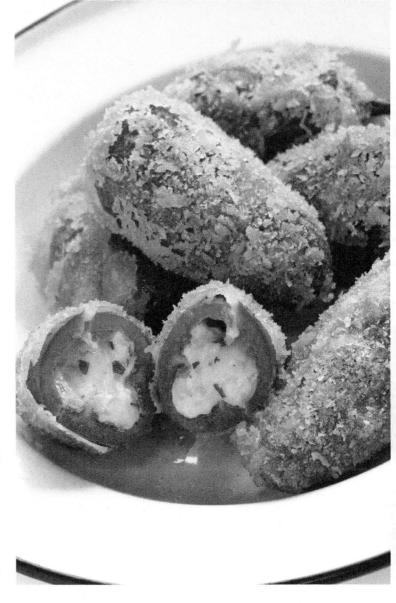

RECOMMENDED ESSENTIAL OILS:

2 drops of sage oil

WHAT YOU WILL NEED:

8 oz. softened cream cheese

1/2 cup Parmesan cheese

12 jalapeños cut in half lengthwise, seeds removed

1/2 cup breadcrumbs

2 eggs, beaten

Splash of milk

1/3 cup flour

Cooking oil

2 tbsp. sage, chopped (or 2 drops sage essential oil)

WHAT TO DO:

1. In a large skillet, add enough cooking oil to cover the jalapenos. Heat the skillet over medium heat.

2. In a large bowl, combine cream cheese and fresh sage (or essential oil). Mix well until the cream cheese is easy to work, then add Parmesan cheese.

3. Take a heaping spoonful of the cheese mixture and stuff the jalapeños.

4. In a shallow bowl, make an egg wash by adding a splash of milk with two beaten eggs.

5. Place the breadcrumbs into a separate dish.

6. Pour flour into a shallow dish, then dip each jalapeño into the flour, then egg wash and then roll them in breadcrumbs.

7. Once the oil is heated, drop a few jalapeños into the oil working in small batches. Cook about 3 minutes per batch. Remove from oil and drain on paper towel. Enjoy!

Chapter 11
Beverages

CITRUS LEMONADE WITH LEMON, ORANGE, TANGERINE, GRAPEFRUIT AND GINGER OIL

Serves 4-6

Wake up your senses with this combination of fresh fruit juice in a delicious spritzer.

RECOMMENDED ESSENTIAL OILS:

- 1 drop of lemon oil
- 1 drop of orange oil
- 1 drop of tangerine oil
- 1 drop of grapefruit oil
- 1 drop of ginger oil

WHAT YOU WILL NEED:

- 3 large oranges
- 1 grapefruit
- 1 lemon
- 1 lime
- Extra fruits slices to add to pitcher or glasses
- Essential oils (your choice)

WHAT TO DO:

1. To make this refreshing spritzer, get all of your fruit out and peel the skin off of each fruit, then process through a juicer.

2. Pour juice into a pitcher, then stir in each drop of essential oil.

3. Finally, add ice and sliced fruit into individual glasses, pour and serve.

 Tip:

After washing fresh fruit or veggies with water, place them in a bowl and toss in a couple of drops of tangerine or lemon essential oil.

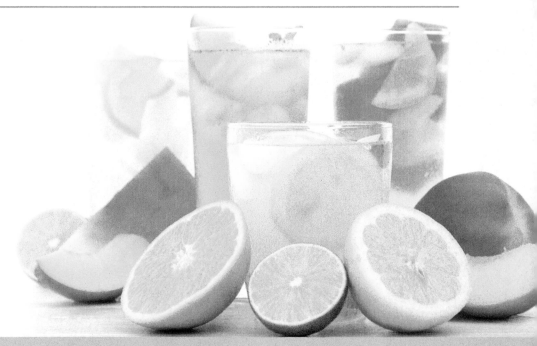

ORANGE SANGRIA WITH ORANGE OIL

Serves 6-8

This is a beautiful presentation of a sweet and delicious fruit sangria infused with flavors of oranges, strawberries and apples.

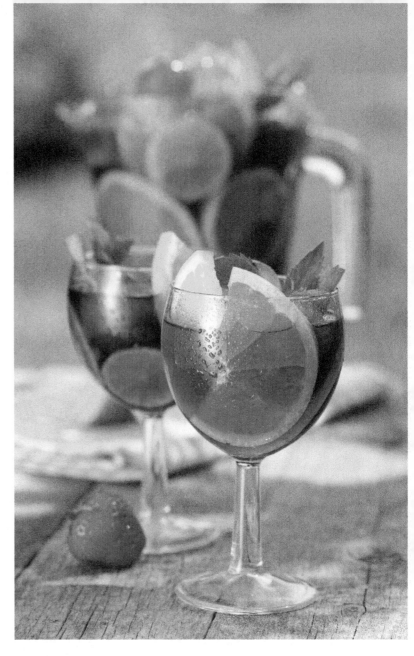

RECOMMENDED ESSENTIAL OILS:

1 drop of orange oil per serving

WHAT YOU WILL NEED:

6 medium-sized oranges, 4 juiced, 2 sliced
2 750 ml bottles of a light white wine
1 cup club soda
1/2 cup Grand Marnier
1 package strawberries, stemmed and sliced
1 red apple, sliced
Sugar to taste

WHAT TO DO:

1. In a pitcher, combine the orange juice, orange slices, wine, Grand Marnier, strawberries and apples. Stir. Place in fridge for 24 hours, allowing the fruits to soak up the sangria.

2. Just before serving, add club soda. Taste test to see if it needs to be sweetened by adding a little sugar.

3. Fill glasses with ice and pour the sangria in. Add one drop of orange oil and fresh slices of fruit to each glass to enhance the presentation.

 Tip:
You may want to add fruit to a toothpick that has been dipped in orange or spearmint essential oil.

SPICED OATMEAL SMOOTHIE WITH CINNAMON AND NUTMEG OIL

Serves 2

Enjoy this tasty smoothie knowing it is heart healthy, too. With a blend of oatmeal, yogurt and spices, you are supplying your body with much needed nutrients that taste great.

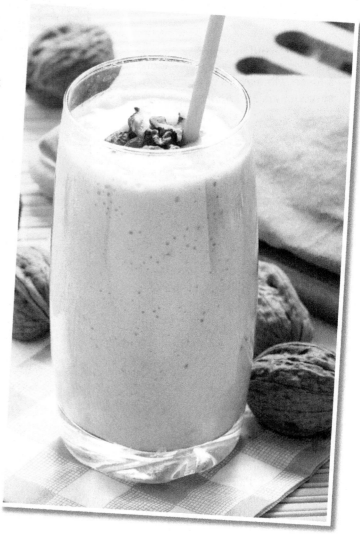

RECOMMENDED ESSENTIAL OILS:

1 drop of cinnamon oil

1 drop of turmeric oil

1 drop of nutmeg oil

WHAT YOU WILL NEED:

1/4 cup quick oats, cooked and cooled

1/2 cup vanilla yogurt

1/2 cup low-fat milk

1 apple peeled, cored and chopped

1 tsp. maple syrup

Pinch of nutmeg (or 1 drop nutmeg essential oil)

½ tsp. ground cinnamon (or 1 drop cinnamon essential oil)

1/8 tsp. ground turmeric (or 1 drop turmeric essential oil)

WHAT TO DO:

1. Combine the oatmeal, milk, yogurt, apple pieces, maple syrup, essential oils or ground spices in a blender and blend well until mixture is smooth and thick.
2. Serve immediately.

 Tip:

For tabouli, add spearmint essential oil using the toothpick method.

KIWI AND APPLE SMOOTHIE WITH LIME OIL

Serves 1

Refresh your taste buds and body when you wake up or enjoy
a mid-afternoon treat with
this chilly kiwi, apple and
lime frozen treat.

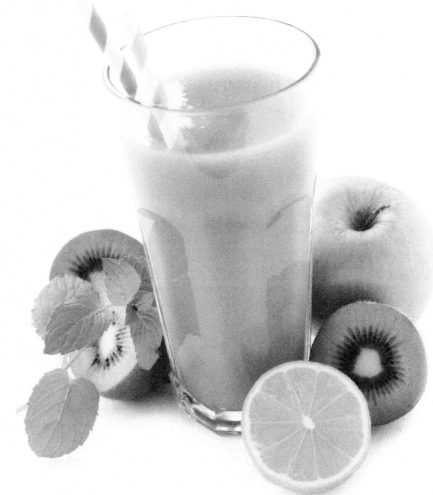

RECOMMENDED ESSENTIAL OILS:

2 drops of lime oil

WHAT YOU WILL NEED:

3 kiwis, chopped

1 apple peeled, cored and cut into pieces

1 handful seedless green grapes

The juice from one fresh lime (or 2 drops lime essential oil)

1/2 cup vanilla yogurt

WHAT TO DO:

1. Add all of the ingredients into a blender and blend until smooth.

2. Serve immediately.

Tip:

For raw foods, essential oils add the most flavor, especially smoothies
and uncooked desserts.

HOT CHOCOLATE WITH PEPPERMINT OIL

Serves 4

A warm glass of hot cocoa with a hint of peppermint is perfect for sipping with those who matter most over the holidays.

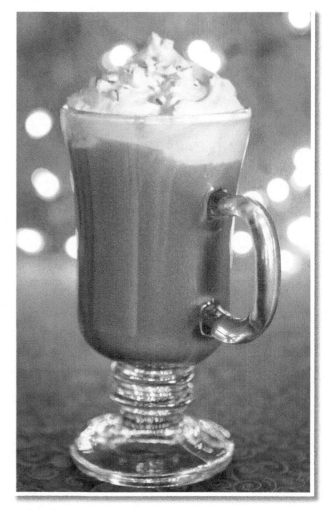

RECOMMENDED ESSENTIAL OILS:

3 drops of peppermint oil

WHAT YOU WILL NEED:

1 1/2 cups heavy cream
1 1/2 cups milk
1/4 cup sugar
Pinch of salt
6 oz. bittersweet chocolate
Whipped cream
Crushed peppermint for topping (optional)
3 drops peppermint essential oil

WHAT TO DO:

1. In a saucepan, add heavy cream, milk, and sugar. Heat on low heat.
2. As soon as the milk is warm, add the chocolate and peppermint essential oil, one drop at a time.
3. Stir frequently until the chocolate is melted. Top with whipped cream and serve.

 Tip:
Place fresh mint or a drop of peppermint essential oil in the bottom of a cup of hot chocolate for a cool and refreshing taste.

CHAMOMILE ICED TEA WITH LAVENDER AND SPEARMINT OIL

Serves 8-10

This light and refreshing chamomile iced tea that you can infuse with lavender and spearmint flavors is great for a relaxing afternoon.

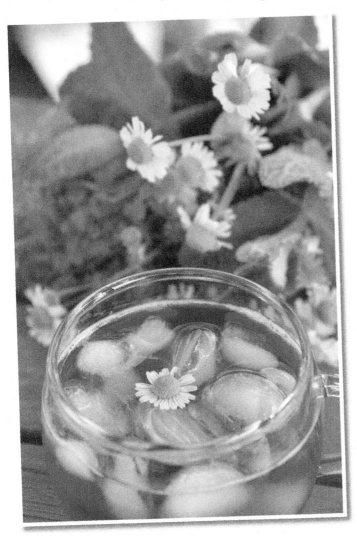

RECOMMENDED ESSENTIAL OILS:

2 drops of lavender oil
4 drops of spearmint oil

WHAT YOU WILL NEED:

2 tbsp. dried culinary lavender
1 cup crushed mint
4 chamomile tea bags
Water
2 drops lavender essential oil
4 drops spearmint essential oil

WHAT TO DO:

1. Take a one-gallon drink storage container and muddle the mint in the bottom, if you are using leaves. Place chamomile tea bags in the bottom. Pour in boiling water to fill 3/4 of the container.

2. Steep until the mixture becomes room temperature. Remove the tea bags, then add the lavender and/or mint oils. Stir.

3. Store in the refrigerator and serve over ice straining out the herbs when pouring into glasses.

Tip:
Make hot or cold teas by adding two drops of lavender, roman chamomile, orange, lemon, or peppermint with a teaspoon of honey and stir into a cup of warm water.

Chapter 12
Soups

FRENCH ONION SOUP WITH ONION OIL

Serves 4

Enjoy this heartwarming bowl of melted Swiss cheese covering caramelized onions in a beef stock.

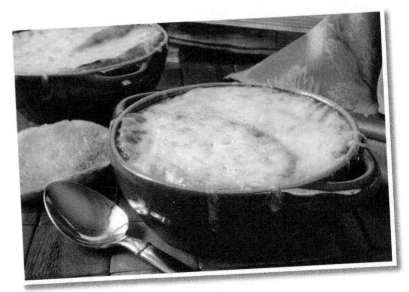

RECOMMENDED ESSENTIAL OILS:

2 drops of onion oil

WHAT YOU WILL NEED:

1/4 cup butter

2 lbs. onions

2 lbs. yellow onions, sliced

2 tsp. granulated sugar

1 heaping tbsp. flour

3 1/2 cup beef stock

2 cups filtered water

1/4 cup cognac

1 1/2 tsp. sea salt

1/2 tsp. ground black pepper

1 loaf French bread (sliced into pieces about 3/4 in. thick)

1 1/2 lbs. Swiss cheese
(and 2 drops onion essential oil)

WHAT TO DO:

1. In a large skillet, melt the butter.
2. Add in the onion and sugar then cover, allowing them to soften and lightly brown over low to medium heat.
3. Remove the lid and continue to cook the onions for about 20 minutes more so that they caramelize. Be careful not to burn them.
4. Preheat oven to 400 degrees. Once the onions are done, add in the flour and combine it well, followed by the water, 3 tablespoons of cognac, onion essential oil, salt and pepper. After about 10 minutes of simmering, add in the rest of the cognac.
5. Place sliced bread in the oven and toast for approximately 5 minutes per side.
6. Divide the soup into four bowls and place slices of bread in each bowl. Cover each bowl with slices of Swiss cheese and to broil.
7. Place the bowls on a cookie sheet and insert in the oven to melt the cheese. Remove with done. Be sure to warn everyone the bowls are hot!

TOMATO SOUP WITH BASIL OIL

Serves 2

Whether you make quesadillas, grilled cheese or croutons, this soup will go with them perfectly. The classic blend of tomatoes and herbs makes for a heartwarming meal.

RECOMMENDED ESSENTIAL OILS:

1 drop of basil oil
1 drop of garlic oil

WHAT YOU WILL NEED:

6 Roma tomatoes
1/2 tsp. fresh oregano, chopped
2 sun-dried tomatoes
1/4 tsp. ground black pepper
1/2 tsp. sea salt
1/2 tsp. fresh basil (or 1 drop basil essential oil)
1 garlic clove (or 1 drop garlic essential oil)
Water
Basil leaves for garnishing

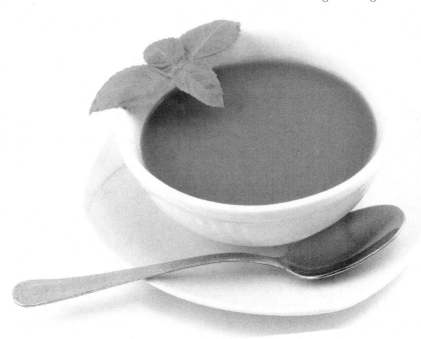

WHAT TO DO:

1. In a food processor, pulse the tomatoes until smooth. Add water in until you have the consistency that you want.

2. Peel the skin off the garlic clove and drop into the processor (or add one drop of garlic oil and one drop of basil oil). Pulse.

3. Add in the sun-dried tomatoes, salt and pepper. Once smooth pour into a saucepan and heat thoroughly over medium heat, careful not to burn.

4. Serve immediately. Opt to make this dish pretty with a leaf of basil.

CHICKEN NOODLE SOUP WITH THYME AND PARSLEY OIL

Serves 8-12

There is nothing more comforting than a warm steaming bowl of chicken noodle soup. Enjoy this variation rounded out with the flavors of parsley and thyme.

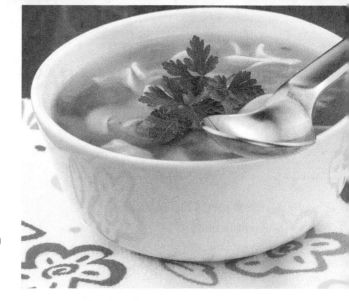

RECOMMENDED ESSENTIAL OILS:

1 drop of thyme oil

1 drop of parsley oil

WHAT YOU WILL NEED:

3 1/2 lbs. chicken (cut into parts)

2 carrots (cleaned, not peeled and sliced in 2 in. pieces for stock)

3 carrots (peel and cut into 1/4-in. rounds for soup)

2 ribs celery (cut into 2 in. slices for stock)

3 ribs celery (cut into 1/4-in. slices for soup)

1 onion (quartered, for stock)

3 garlic cloves, peeled and halved

5 peppercorns

Salt to taste

8-12 oz. egg noodles

1 tbsp. dried thyme (or 1 drop thyme essential oil)

1 tbsp. dried parsley (or 1 drop parsley essential oil)

Freshly ground black pepper to taste

WHAT TO DO:

1. Start by removing the breast and thigh meat from the respective bones. Put in a bowl, cover and place in the refrigerator to chill until needed for preparing the soup. Discard the skin. Next, remove and discard excess fat from the chicken pieces.

2. In a large pot, add in breast and thigh bones, the back, legs, neck and wings. Cover the pot with water and bring to a boil for about 5 minutes (skimming away and discarding the scum that comes to the surface). Once boiled, remove it from the heat, drain off the water and rinse the bones and the pot.

3. Return the parboiled bones into the cleaned pot. Add in the 2-inch sliced carrots and celery ribs and some celery tops if you have them. Leek greens or fennel tops can be added, too (optional).

4. Next, add in the onion, garlic cloves, thyme (oil or dried herbs), parsley (oil or dried herbs) and peppercorns.

5. Cover the pot with about 3 quarts of water and bring to a low simmer (about 185 degrees). Let it simmer, partially covered, for about 1 1/2 hours until the stock is just barely bubbling. After 1 1/2 hours, strain out the bones and vegetables, reserving the stock. If you want, set aside and strip the bones of any remaining meat.

6. Rinse out the pot and return the stock to the pot. Taste the stock and season to taste.

7. For 3 quarts of stock you can add 2 tablespoons of salt. Add the sliced carrots and celery to the stock and bring it to a simmer.

8. Next, slice the chicken breast and thigh meat into bite-sized pieces and add to the pot.

9. Add in the egg noodles and return to a simmer. Simmer for about 5 minutes or until the egg noodles are just barely cooked and the chicken is just cooked through.

10. Lastly, stir in a handful of chopped fresh parsley, freshly ground black pepper, some thyme and salt to taste.

SAUSAGE GUMBO WITH BAY LEAF, THYME AND PARSLEY OIL

Serves 6-8

When you want a rich and filling meal that is full of flavor, gumbo is the way to go. Enjoy this gumbo filled with herbs, vegetables spices and flavorful sausage.

RECOMMENDED ESSENTIAL OILS:

1 drop of bay leaf oil

1 drop of thyme oil

1 drop of parsley oil

WHAT YOU WILL NEED:

4 tbsp. bacon fat

4 tbsp. flour

1 onion, diced

4 cloves garlic, minced

4-6 cups simmering chicken stock

29 oz. whole peeled tomatoes

1 medium green pepper, chopped

2 ribs celery, chopped

4 cups fresh okra, chopped

1-2 bay leaves (optional)

1 tbsp. dried thyme (or 1 drop thyme essential oil)

1 tbsp. dried parsley (or 1 drop parsley essential oil)

2 bay leaves (or 1 drop bay leaf essential oil)

Salt and pepper

2 lb. Andouille sausage, sliced

2 cups rice

WHAT TO DO:

1. Start by mixing the bacon fat and the flour in a large heavy pot. Sauté it on medium-low heat until it becomes brown, stirring frequently. When it is finally dark brown and shiny (if it is dried and powdered it is burnt!), add in the onion and cook again for about 15 minutes or until the onions caramelize and turn translucent, stirring frequently.

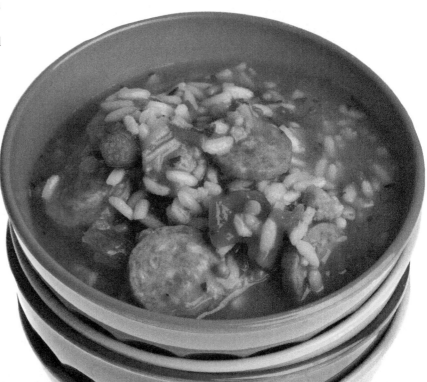

2. Next, add in the garlic and cook for about 1 to 2 minutes followed by the chicken stock. Now, pour the chicken stock in slowly, while stirring.

3. Add in chopped vegetables, tomatoes, bay leaf (or bay leaf essential oil), thyme (or thyme essential oil), parsley (or parsley essential oil), celery leaves, salt and pepper to taste.

4. Cook on medium heat for about 30 minutes or until the vegetables are tender.

5. Add the sausage and cook over medium heat until heated thoroughly. Continue stirring.

6. Finally, sprinkle the top with chopped green onions. Transfer to serving bowls and serve.

BROCCOLI CHEESE SOUP WITH TARRAGON OIL

Serves 6

RECOMMENDED ESSENTIAL OILS:

1 drop of tarragon oil

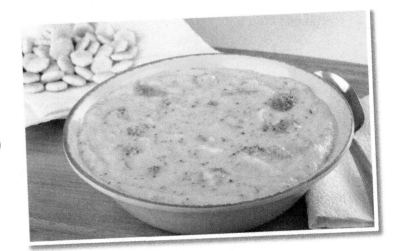

WHAT YOU WILL NEED:

6 tbsp. butter (at room temperature)

2 lbs. broccoli, chopped

1 yellow onion, diced

2 garlic cloves, minced

6 1/2 cups chicken stock

1 cup whipping cream

3 tbsp. all-purpose flour

8 oz. extra-sharp cheddar cheese, grated

1 tsp. fresh tarragon (or 1 drop tarragon essential oil)

WHAT TO DO:

1. In a medium pot, melt 3 tablespoons of butter over medium-high heat.

2. Add in the broccoli stems and onions; sauté them for about 6 minutes or until the onions are softened.

3. Next, add in the garlic and tarragon (if using tarragon oil, dip a toothpick in the oil and stir it into the mixture); sauté again for 1 minute.

4. Stir in the stock and bring to a boil. Let it simmer uncovered for about 15 minutes or until the broccoli is tender.

5. Pour in the cream.

6. In a small bowl, mix the remaining 3 tablespoons of butter with the flour to make a paste. Whisk that paste into the soup.

7. Now it is time for the broccoli. Add in broccoli pieces and simmer them for about 5 minutes. The soup will thicken as the broccoli becomes tender; stir frequently.

8. Refrigerate several hours to meld the flavors.

9. When ready to eat, remove from the fridge and warm again. Preheat the broiler and place 6 ovenproof soup bowls on baking sheet.

10. Add the soup into the serving bowls and top each with 1/3 cup of cheese. Broil for about 4 minutes until the cheese melts and bubbles around edges. Serve and enjoy.

SPICY CHILI WITH BAY LEAF, GARLIC AND OREGANO OIL

Serves 6

When it's cold outside, this chili is the perfect anecdote to create a warm home that is filled with a southwestern aroma.

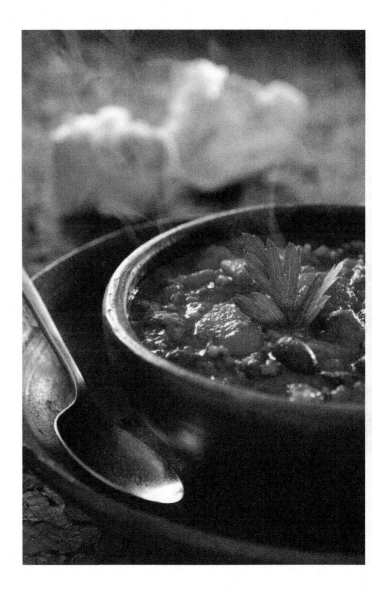

RECOMMENDED ESSENTIAL OILS:

1 drop of bay leaf oil

1 drop of oregano oil

2 drops of garlic oil

WHAT YOU WILL NEED:

6 oz. turkey sausage (hot)

2 cups onions, chopped

1 cup green bell pepper, chopped

1 lb. ground sirloin

1 jalapeno, chopped

2 tbsp. chili powder

2 tbsp. brown sugar

1 tbsp. ground cumin

3 tbsp. tomato paste

1/2 tsp. fresh pepper

1/4 tsp. salt

1 1/4 cups merlot

28 oz. whole tomatoes, coarsely chopped

15 oz. kidney beans, drained

2 bay leaves (or 1 drop bay leaf essential oil)

1 tsp. dried oregano (or 1 drop oregano essential oil)

8 garlic cloves, minced (or 2 drops garlic essential oil)

2 oz. shredded cheddar cheese

WHAT TO DO:

1. Preheat a large Dutch oven over medium-high heat.

2. Remove any casing on the sausage and break up the meat. Add sausage and the chopped onions to the Dutch oven.

3. Next, add the bell pepper, ground sirloin, jalapeno and minced garlic (or garlic essential oil). Sauté until the meat is browned and starts to crumble.

4. Stir in the chili powder, brown sugar, cumin, tomato paste, pepper, salt, dried oregano (or oregano oil using the toothpick method) and two bay leaves (or bay leaf oil using the toothpick method).

5. Combine well. Next, add in the wine, beans and tomatoes.

6. Bring the chili to a boil then reduce heat and cover. Allow to simmer for an hour while periodically stirring it.

7. Uncover the pot for the last 30 minutes, stirring occasionally. When ready to serve, pour into bowls and sprinkle cheese on top.

Tip:

Did you know adding 3 stalks of celery (chopped) to a pot of beans makes the dish easier to digest?

Chapter 13
Salads

CHINESE CHICKEN SALAD WITH CILANTRO AND GINGER OIL

Serves 4

If you are in the mood for a delicious twist on a Chinese chicken salad, this salad spices it up with bell peppers and a dressing loaded with flavor.

RECOMMENDED ESSENTIAL OILS:

1 drop of ginger oil

1 drop of cilantro (or coriander) essential oil

WHAT YOU WILL NEED:

1 lb. chicken breast (cut into strips)

1 tbsp. sesame oil

1 tbsp. canola oil

1/2 tsp. red pepper flakes

1 head iceberg lettuce, sliced

1/2 sweet bell pepper, sliced

3-4 sliced scallions

1 carrot cut into sticks

1/2 cup loosely packed cilantro leaves, chopped

1/2 cup roasted peanuts

Salt to taste

Chow mein noodles

FOR THE DRESSING:

1 tbsp. soy sauce

2 tbsp. rice vinegar

1 tsp. mustard powder

1 garlic clove, minced

1/2 tsp. chili pepper flakes

2 tsp. sugar

1 tbsp. dark sesame oil

1/4 cup canola oil

1 tsp. fresh ginger (or 1 drop ginger essential oil)

4 tbsp. fresh cilantro (or 1 drop cilantro or coriander essential oil)

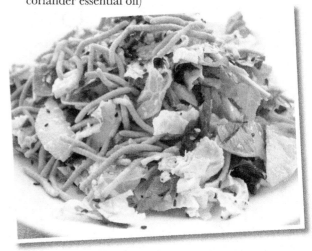

WHAT TO DO:

1. In a large saucepan, heat the canola and sesame oils over high heat for 1 minute.

2. Add in red pepper flakes and cook them for 30 seconds.

3. Season the chicken strips with a little salt and add them into the pan. Stir and sauté the chicken on high heat for 3 to 6 minutes or until browned. Remove the chicken and set it on a plate to the side.

4. For the dressing, in a small bowl whisk the dressing ingredients together and season with salt and pepper to taste. Remember you can use a drop of ginger essential oil or cilantro essential oil in place of fresh herbs.

5. In a large bowl, toss together the chicken with the lettuce, bell pepper, cilantro, scallions, carrots and peanuts.

6. Just before serving, toss salad with dressing and top with the chow mein noodles.

PEAR AND WALNUT SALAD WITH CINNAMON, NUTMEG, CARDAMOM AND VANILLA OIL

Serves 1

This salad is light and refreshing with crunchy pears and walnuts hiding throughout.

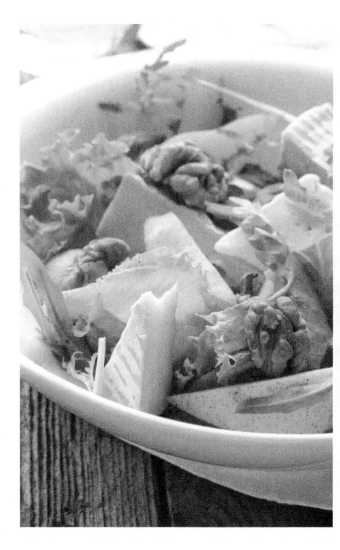

RECOMMENDED ESSENTIAL OILS:

1 drop of cinnamon oil
1 drop of nutmeg oil
1 drop of cardamom oil
1 drop of vanilla oil

WHAT YOU WILL NEED:

2 cups red lettuce leaves (or other colorful lettuce variety)
1/2 cup arugula
1/2 ripe pear
Spiced walnuts
1/4 cup walnuts (halves or pieces)
1 tbsp. raw honey (or 1 dried date + 1 tbsp. water)
1/4 tsp. ground cinnamon (or 1 drop cinnamon essential oil)
1/8 tsp. ground ginger
1/4 tsp. fresh ground nutmeg (or 1 drop nutmeg essential oil)
1/8 tsp. vanilla extract (or 1 drop vanilla essential oil)
1/4 tsp. ground cardamom (or 1 drop cardamom essential oil)

FOR THE DRESSING:

1 orange
2 tbsp. raw apple cider vinegar
2 tsp. sweetener
1 tsp. sesame oil
1 tsp. sesame seeds
1 tsp. ground mustard seeds or whole mustard seeds
1/4 tsp. cracked or ground black pepper

WHAT TO DO:

1. For the salad, rinse, dry and add the lettuce and arugula to a plate.

2. Slice the pear in half and remove seeds.

3. Top the greens with sliced pear.

4. For the walnuts: pour the honey into a bowl and mix in the cinnamon, ginger, nutmeg, vanilla and cardamom. (You can use the ground spices or essential oil drops, or a combination of the two.) Mix well and coat the walnuts in the honey. Sprinkle over the salad.

5. For the dressing, zest and juice the orange.

6. In a food processor, combine orange zest, orange juice, vinegar, sweetener, spices and sesame seeds and process them for about 1 minute, until smooth. Drizzle it on the salad and enjoy!

POTATO SALAD WITH PARSLEY OIL

Serves 6-8

Having a summer barbecue? This potato salad is perfect with bits of bacon mixed into the creamy dressing.

RECOMMENDED ESSENTIAL OILS:

2 drops of parsley oil

3 drops of dill oil

WHAT YOU WILL NEED:

2 lbs. Yukon gold potatoes (cubed into 1 inch cubes)

3/4 cup sour cream

1/4 cup mayonnaise

2 tsp. mustard

2 tbsp. fresh parsley, chopped (or 2 drops parsley essential oil)

1/2 cup green onions, chopped

1/2 cup celery, chopped

1/4 cup parsley, chopped

3/4 cup dill pickles, chopped (or 3 drops dill essential oil)

6 bacon slices, cooked and chopped

Coarse salt to taste

Freshly ground pepper to taste

WHAT TO DO:

1. In a flying pan, add bacon strips in a single layer and cook on medium heat. Brown lightly until most of the fat is cooked out, turning occasionally with tongs.

2. Remove bacon slices and place them on a plate lined with paper towels to soak up the excess fat.

3. In a large pot, add the potatoes and cover them with cold, salted water (about 1 teaspoon salt) and bring to a boil. Reduce heat to low and simmer for about 20 minutes or until the potatoes are tender when poked with a fork.

4. Drain potatoes and rinse with cold water. Add some pickle juice and/or 2-3 drops of dill essential oil to the drained, warm potatoes. The potatoes will soak up the juices, adding great flavor.

5. In a large bowl, whisk together the sour cream, mayonnaise and mustard. Season with salt, pepper, and parsley leaves and/or parsley essential oil.

6. Add the potatoes and combine gently.

7. Add all of the remaining ingredients, combining lightly.

8. Finally, include a couple tablespoons of the pickle juice for good measure. Sprinkle any remaining chopped parsley on top.

Tip:

Dill essential oil makes a wonderful addition to homemade potato salad.

CHEF SALAD AND HOMEMADE RANCH DRESSING WITH DILL AND PARSLEY OIL

Serves 2-3

This classic chef salad is delicious, filling and has a delicious homemade ranch dressing enhanced with dill, oregano, and parsley.

RECOMMENDED ESSENTIAL OILS:

1 drop of dill oil

2 drops of parsley oil

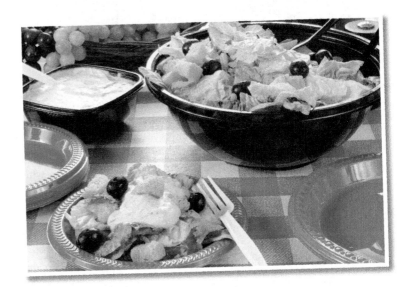

WHAT YOU WILL NEED:

6 cups romaine lettuce, chopped

1/2 lb. bacon, sliced

1/2 lb. oven roasted turkey, sliced

1 tomato, sliced

1 onion, sliced

2 boiled eggs, chopped

1 cup cheddar cheese, shredded

FOR THE RANCH DRESSING:

1-2 garlic cloves

Salt to taste

1/4 cup Italian flat-leaf parsley (or 2 drops parsley essential oil)

2 tbsp. fresh chives

1 cup mayonnaise

1/2 cup sour cream

Buttermilk to taste

White vinegar (optional, to taste)

Fresh dill (optional, to taste)

Cayenne pepper (optional, to taste)

1 tbsp. fresh dill (or 1 drop dill essential oil)

WHAT TO DO:

1. For the dressing, mince the garlic with a knife and sprinkle about 1/4 teaspoon of salt onto it. Mash into a paste with a fork.

2. Finely chop the parsley, chives and any of the optional herbs and add to the garlic.

3. In a bowl, add and combine all ingredients. Add other optional ingredients as needed (taste frequently and adjust seasonings).

4. Add in the parsley and dill essential oils by the drop or by using the toothpick method.

5. Place in the refrigerator for 2 to 3 hours to chill before serving. Stir in milk or buttermilk, if desired, to obtain desired consistency.

6. Divide your lettuce on the plates and top it with sliced tomatoes, chopped eggs, turkey, bacon, onions, cheese and the ranch dressing.

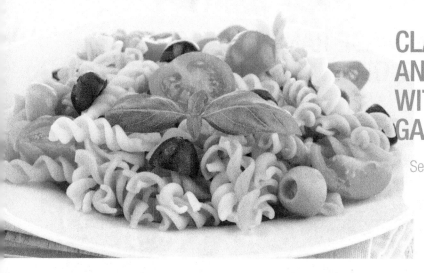

CLASSIC PASTA SALAD AND ITALIAN DRESSING WITH THYME, OREGANO, GARLIC AND ONION OIL

Serves 6-8

Bring this pasta salad to a potluck and it will surely be a favorite. It is easy to whip up for a group of people.

RECOMMENDED ESSENTIAL OILS:

1 drop of thyme oil
1 drop of oregano oil
1 drop of onion oil
1 drop of garlic oil

WHAT YOU WILL NEED:

1 box tri-color rotini pasta
¼ cup black olives, halved
½ cup green olives
½ cup Roma tomatoes, sliced
½ cup feta cheese (optional)

FOR THE ITALIAN DRESSING:

(Makes approximately 2 cups of dressing)
1 cup white wine vinegar
1 1/3 cups extra-virgin olive oil
2 tbsp. water
1/2 tbsp. garlic powder (or 1 drop garlic essential oil)
1/2 tbsp. onion powder (or 1 drop onion essential oil)
1 tbsp. dried oregano (or 1 drop oregano essential oil)
1/2 tbsp. sugar
1/2 tsp. freshly ground black pepper
1/2 tbsp. + 1/2 tsp. Italian seasoning
1/4 tsp. dried thyme (or 1 drop thyme essential oil)
1 tbsp. salt

WHAT TO DO:

1. In a medium-sized bowl, add in the garlic powder (or essential oil), onion powder (or essential oil), oregano leaves (or essential oil), thyme leaves (or essential oil), sugar, pepper, Italian seasoning, and salt. Whisk together to combine flavors.

2. Stir in vinegar, olive oil, and water.

3. Transfer the dressing into a jar or container with a sealable lid. Place the lid on the container and store in the refrigerator for 2 hours.

4. For the pasta, boil water and cook according to package directions.

5. Drain and set aside to cool. Once cooled, move the pasta into a large bowl to add all the other ingredients; add in the tomatoes, olives and Italian dressing.

6. Smoothly toss to coat pasta with the dressing and evenly distribute the chopped veggies. Add remaining dressing mixture and mix well.

7. Place salad into the refrigerator for about 30 minutes to allow flavors to meld. Remove and serve cold or at room temperature.

CHICKEN SALAD WITH TARRAGON OIL

Serves 4-6

This creamy chicken salad has hints of sweet cranberries, apples and onions and tastes great all by itself or on a sandwich.

RECOMMENDED ESSENTIAL OILS:

2 drops of tarragon oil

WHAT YOU WILL NEED:

2 cups cooked chicken, diced

1 small green apple (cored and diced about 1 1/2 cups)

1/3 cup celery, diced

1/3 cup cranberries

1/4 cup red onions, diced

3/4 cup mayonnaise

1 tbsp. fresh lemon juice

1 tbsp. fresh parsley leaves, chopped

1 tbsp. fresh chives, chopped

1/4 tsp. kosher salt

1/4 tsp. freshly ground black pepper

2 tbsp. tarragon leaves, chopped (or 2 drops tarragon essential oil)

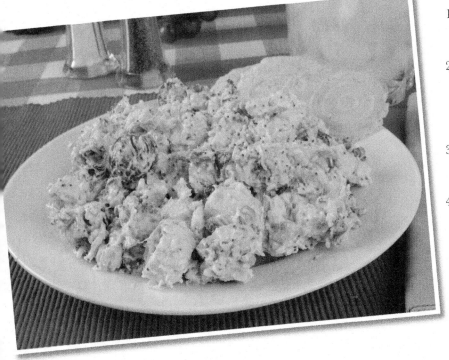

WHAT TO DO:

1. In a medium bowl, add and mix the chicken, apple, celery and onions together.

2. In a another bowl, mix the mayonnaise, lemon juice, parsley, tarragon (oil or leaves), cranberries, chives, salt and pepper.

3. Pour the dressing over the chicken mixture and stir to combine well.

4. Place into the refrigerator for at least 1 hour before serving.

Chapter 14
Vegetables

BACON WRAPPED ASPARAGUS WITH BLACK PEPPER OIL

Servings are adjustable as needed

Everything is better with bacon, and these asparagus spears are no exception. Taste these flavors with a hint of black pepper.

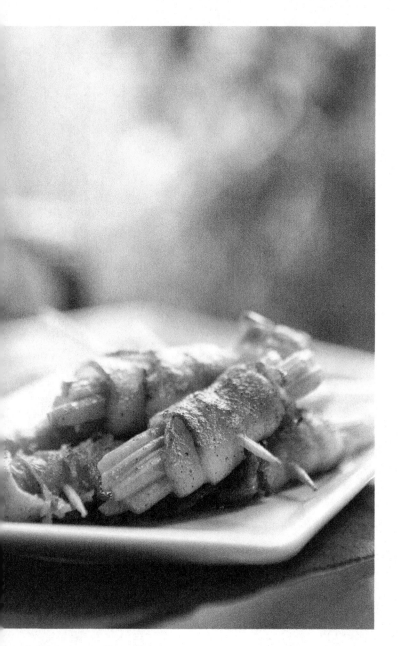

RECOMMENDED ESSENTIAL OILS:

1 drop of black pepper oil

WHAT YOU WILL NEED:

Smoked bacon

Asparagus

Olive oil

1 tbsp. ground black pepper (or 1 drop black pepper essential oil)

WHAT TO DO:

1. Trim and remove the asparagus spear's woody ends, then cut into 1-inch pieces.
2. Mix together 1 tablespoon of black pepper or 1 drop of essential oil with 4 tablespoon of olive oil and brush the mixture over the asparagus.
3. Next, slice the strips of bacon in half. Then, wrap each piece of asparagus in the bacon and thread onto skewers.
4. Grill the skewers for about 5 to 6 minutes, flip and grill again for another 5 minutes or until the asparagus is tender and the bacon is crisp.
5. Sprinkle with freshly ground black pepper and salt before serving.

GLAZED CARROTS WITH ORANGE AND BASIL OIL

Serves 4

These carrots are a perfect side dish to add a splash of color and flavor to a meal.

RECOMMENDED ESSENTIAL OILS:

1 drop of basil oil
2 drops of orange oil

WHAT YOU WILL NEED:

1 lb. carrots
1 cup orange juice (or 2 drops orange
essential oil)
1/4 tsp. salt
1/2 tsp. dried basil (or 1 drop basil essential oil)
Ground black pepper to taste

WHAT TO DO:

1. Fill a large pot half full with water and bring to a boil.

2. Rinse, peel and slice the carrots into 1/4-inch slices.

3. Then, in a medium skillet, heat the orange juice over medium heat until it thickens and reduces by about 3/4. Be careful after it reduces by 1/2, so that it does not boil dry in the pan. The juice will take about 20 minutes to reduce down.

4. Add the carrots into the boiling water. Cook them for about 7 to 10 minutes until slightly soft, but still a bit crunchy. Drain the carrots and rinse under cold water.

5. In a medium bowl, add the orange juice sauce and 1-2 drops of orange essential oil. Stir in basil oil, using the toothpick method. Add basil leaves, if desired.

6. Add in the carrots, salt and black pepper. Toss together well until the carrots are fully coated.

7. Add in any other seasonings according to your liking.

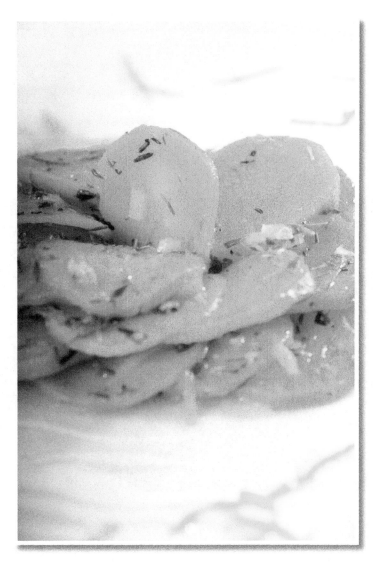

HERB AND GOAT CHEESE STUFFED BELL PEPPERS WITH MARJORAM OIL

Serves 6-8

The creamy goat cheese freckled with a variety of herbs gives a creamy filling to the roasted bell peppers.

RECOMMENDED ESSENTIAL OILS:

2 drops of marjoram oil

2 drops of basil oil

WHAT YOU WILL NEED:

8 small bell peppers

2 tbsp. olive oil

Pinch of salt

Pinch of pepper

11 oz. goat cheese

3-4 tbsp. herb mix (marjoram, basil, chives)

Balsamic glaze

2 tbsp. fresh or dried marjoram (or 2 drops marjoram essential oil)

2 tsp. fresh or dried basil leaves (or 2 drops basil essential oil)

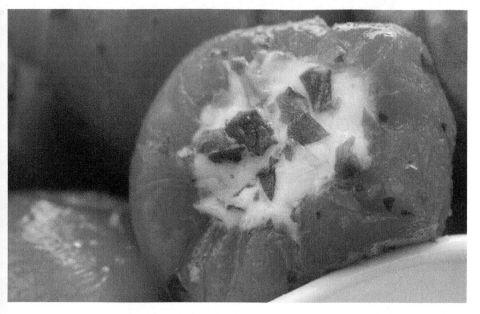

WHAT TO DO:

1. Preheat the oven to 450 degrees.

2. Make a small slit down the center of the peppers. Rinse them and clean the inside out. Remove any seeds.

3. In a bowl, mix the goat cheese, herbs or essential oils, salt and pepper until smooth.

4. Stuff each pepper with the goat cheese mixture and drizzle the tops of the peppers with olive oil.

5. Place in the oven and roast for about 15 to 20 minutes or until cheese is melted and peppers are soft.

6. Remove and lightly drizzle balsamic glaze over each pepper. (Remember, do not use too much balsamic glaze as it is a strong flavor.) Serve warm.

SAUTÉED MUSHROOMS WITH LEMON, THYME AND GARLIC OIL

Serves 3-4

Mushrooms are a canvas that can present anything. In this creamy dish mushrooms take on garlic, thyme, lemon, and of course, butter.

RECOMMENDED ESSENTIAL OILS:

1 drop of garlic oil
1 drop of thyme oil
2 drops of lemon oil

WHAT YOU WILL NEED:

3 tbsp. olive oil
10 oz. fresh white mushrooms or button-mushrooms (slice the big ones into thick slices and keep the small ones whole)
1 tbsp. unsalted butter
Sea salt
Freshly ground black pepper

1/4 cup dry white wine
½ tbsp. fresh flat-leaf parsley + more to garnish, chopped
2 tsp. lemon juice (or 2 drops lemon essential oil)
½ tbsp. minced garlic (or 1 drop garlic essential oil)
½ tsp. fresh thyme, minced (or 1 drop thyme essential oil)

WHAT TO DO:

1. In a large skillet, add the olive oil and warm on medium-high heat. Once the oil is hot, sprinkle the mushrooms in a single layer across it.

2. Allow them to sizzle for about 2 minutes or until they caramelize on the bottom (if you toss them too soon, they will release their liquid and start to steam).

3. Once the bottoms are caramelized, toss and cook on high for five minutes. Drain off excess oil and discard.

4. While the mushrooms are still in the skillet, stir in the garlic, thyme and lemon essential oils into the butter, then pour over the mushrooms. Continue to cook for 2-3 minutes until mushrooms are beautifully brown, stirring occasionally.

5. Season with salt and pepper to taste and add the minced garlic if you are using it. Sauté again for about 2 minutes or until the garlic is lightly browned.

6. Next, add in the wine. Slightly reduce heat, and simmer the mushrooms until they are glazed with the sauce.

7. Lastly, add in the parsley then transfer to a warmed bowl and serve immediately.

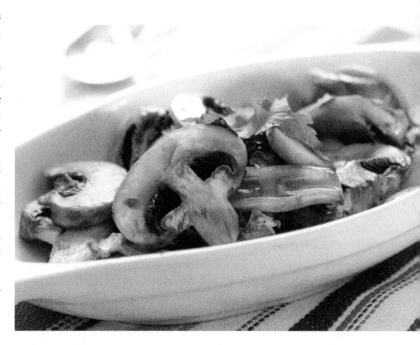

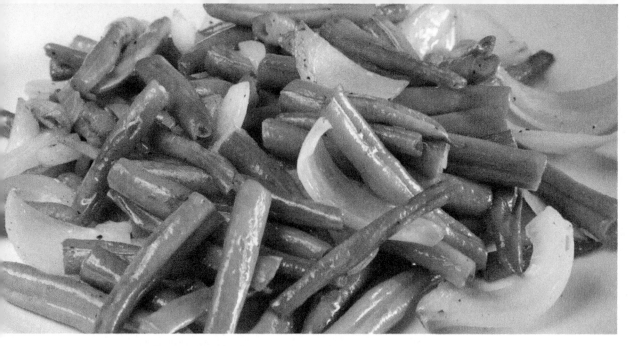

SAUTÉED GREEN BEANS WITH CUMIN AND SAFFRON OIL

Serves 4

Try a new flavor with your green beans by combining shallots, cumin and saffron into the mix.

RECOMMENDED ESSENTIAL OILS:

1 drop of saffron oil
1 drop of cumin seed oil

WHAT YOU WILL NEED:

1 lb. green beans, cleaned and trimmed
1 tbsp. olive oil
1 shallot, thinly sliced
1/4 tsp. kosher salt
1/2 cup water
1 tsp. sherry vinegar
1 pinch Saffron (or 1 drop saffron essential oil)
½ tsp. ground cumin seed (or 1 drop cumin seed essential oil)

WHAT TO DO:

1. Combine the cumin oil with the olive oil and heat it in a large saucepan over medium heat.

2. Add in the shallots and sauté them for a few minutes until they soften.

3. Next, add the green beans and stir to coat the beans fully with the oil and cumin, and sauté again for a few minutes. If you are using saffron, crumble the saffron on the green beans and sprinkle with the salt. If you are using saffron oil, add oil into water using the toothpick method, then pour water to the saucepan. Cover and steam for about 5 minutes or until the green beans are tender.

4. Remove cover and allow any water still in the pan to evaporate.

5. Remove pan from heat and sprinkle the vinegar over the green beans. Stir well. Serve immediately hot or at room temperature.

PICKLED CUCUMBERS WITH CELERY SEED OIL

Serves 10

Make your own pickles using celery seed oil and a few mason jars!

RECOMMENDED ESSENTIAL OILS:

1 drop of celery seed oil

WHAT YOU WILL NEED:

7 cups cucumbers, peeled and sliced

1 tsp. salt

2 cups granulated sugar

1 cup red onion, chopped

1 cup green bell pepper, chopped

1 cup cider vinegar

1 tsp. celery seed (or 1 drop celery seed essential oil)

WHAT TO DO:

1. In a mixing bowl, add and mix the cucumbers with the salt and let sit for about 1 hour.

2. Don't drain the mixture; add in the sugar, onions, bell pepper, cider vinegar and celery seed.

3. If using essential oil dip the toothpick in the celery seed oil then mix it into the bowl. Mix well, cover and then place into the refrigerator. You can add more herbs of your liking if you choose. Enjoy!

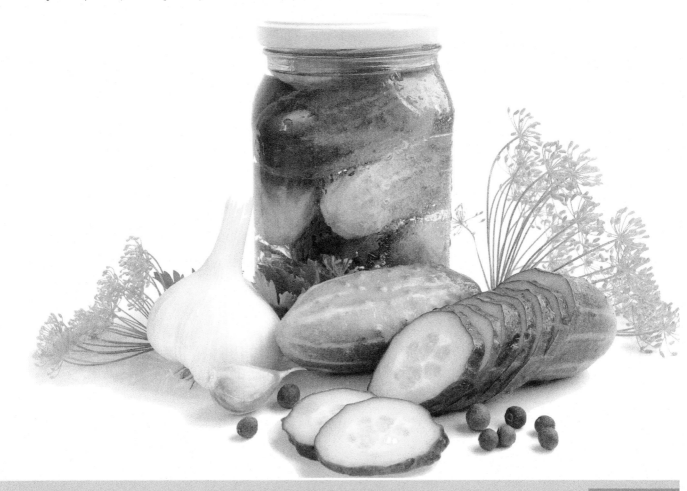

Chapter 15
Side Dishes

BAKED MACARONI AND CHEESE WITH ROSEMARY AND THYME OIL

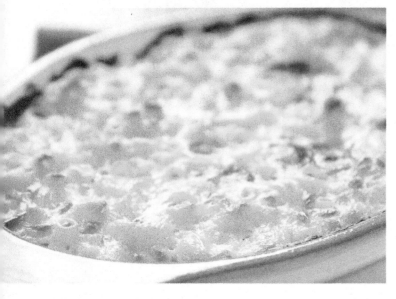

Serves 3-4

Home cooking like only Mama does! This macaroni and cheese is baked to crispy perfection.

RECOMMENDED ESSENTIAL OILS:

1 drop of rosemary oil
1 drop of thyme oil

WHAT YOU WILL NEED:

9 oz. macaroni
1 1/2 oz. butter
1 1/2 oz. flour
1 pint milk
2 oz. breadcrumbs
3 oz. herbs

9 oz. cheddar cheese, grated
2 oz. parmesan, grated
Salt to taste
Pepper to taste
1 tsp. dried rosemary (or 1 drop rosemary essential oil)
1 tsp. dried thyme (or 1 drop thyme essential oil)

WHAT TO DO:

1. Preheat oven to 200 degrees.

2. Boil the macaroni in a large pot on the stove top. Once the water has reached a boil, turn the heat down to a low and simmer for about 10 to 12 minutes or until the pasta is cooked through, but still has a slight toughness.

3. Remove the pot from the heat and drain macaroni well using a colander.

4. In another small pan, melt the butter on medium heat.

5. Stir in flour to make a roux. Slowly add the milk, stirring continuously until all the milk is used and you get a thick, pourable white sauce.

6. Next, add in the chopped herbs or stir in essential oils using the toothpick method. Add in grated cheddar cheese and parmesan (reserve a little of both for topping) and stir until well combined.

7. Mix the cheese sauce in with the macaroni and season it to taste.

8. Pour the macaroni cheese into the microwave safe dish and top with the leftover cheese, salt, pepper and the breadcrumbs.

9. Place pan in an oven about 12 to 15 minutes or until the top is golden brown. Remove and enjoy.

HERBED CHEESY MASHED POTATOES WITH DILL OIL

Serves 6-8

Not your average mashed potatoes! These potatoes have a hint of chives, basil and dill along with sautéed scallion, cheese and butter which combine to make a flavorful dish.

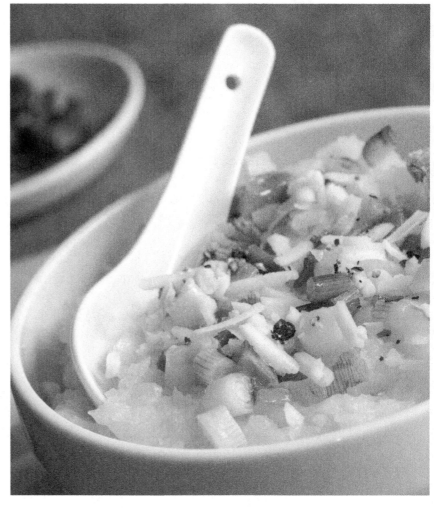

RECOMMENDED ESSENTIAL OILS:

1 drop of dill oil

WHAT YOU WILL NEED:

3 lbs. yellow potatoes
1/4 cup unsalted butter
3/4 cup scallions, sliced
1 tbsp. chopped fresh or 1 tsp. dried basil
1 tbsp. chopped fresh or 1 tsp. dried chives
1 tsp. salt
1/2 tsp. black pepper
1 1/2 cups mild cheddar cheese, shredded
1/2 cup milk
1 tsp. dried dill (or 1 drop dill essential oil)

WHAT TO DO:

1. In a large pot, boil the potatoes until they are soft. This should take about 20-25 minutes.

2. In another saucepan, melt butter over medium heat.

3. Add in the scallions and sauté for about one minute.

4. Turn heat to low, then stir in salt, pepper, chives, basil and dried dill (or dill essential oil using the toothpick method).

5. Drain the potatoes and rinse the pot, then add them back in. Mix the scallions in well with the potatoes.

6. Add in the cheese and milk and beat until smooth.

7. Top with sliced chives and scallions.

MIXED HERB RICE PILAF WITH PARSLEY, TARRAGON AND BASIL OIL

Serves 6-8

A flavorful pilaf, enhanced with parsley, tarragon and basil that goes perfect with fish or chicken entrees.

RECOMMENDED ESSENTIAL OILS:

1 drop of parsley oil
1 drop of tarragon oil
2 drops of basil oil

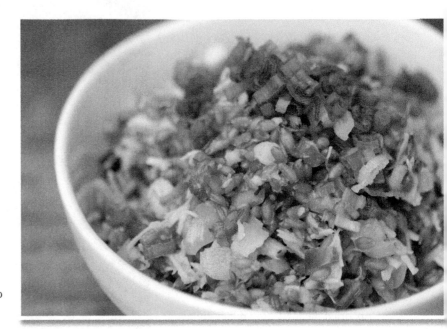

WHAT YOU WILL NEED:

1/4 cup olive oil
1/2 cup yellow onions, diced
1 tsp. garlic, minced
2 cups long grain rice
2 tsp. salt
1 tsp. pepper
3 cups chicken broth
2 tbsp. fresh parsley (or 1 drop parsley essential oil)
2 tbsp. fresh tarragon (or 1 drop tarragon essential oil)
4 tbsp. fresh basil (or 2 drops basil essential oil)

WHAT TO DO:

1. Using a 2-quart saucepan, add olive oil and heat it over medium-high heat.

2. Sauté the onions in the pan until they soften and become translucent.

3. Add in the minced garlic and stir for about 45 seconds. If you have the essential oils, add them in at this point. If you are using herbs, wait until the end.

4. Add the rice and be sure to mix in well with the onions and garlic. Allow to toast for about 5 minutes.

5. Add salt and pepper, followed by the chicken stock.

6. Bring the mixture to a boil, then place the cover on the pan.

7. Slide it into the oven and let sit for 30 minutes. When ready, top with any remaining fresh herbs and serve.

HEARTY STUFFING WITH THYME AND SAGE OIL

Serves 8

It doesn't have to be Thanksgiving to enjoy this side dish favorite. Find surprises in each bite whether it's mushrooms, cornbread, pecans or celery bites.

RECOMMENDED ESSENTIAL OILS:

1 drop of thyme oil
1 drop of sage oil

WHAT YOU WILL NEED:

12 oz. sausage, chopped
1/2 cup butter
3 cups onion, diced
1 cup celery, chopped
3 cups sliced mushrooms
6 cups cornbread, crumbled
6 cups white bread, crumbled
1 tbsp. poultry seasoning

1 tsp. salt
1 tsp. black pepper
1 cup pecans
1 1/2 cups chicken broth
2 eggs
1 tsp. dried sage (or 1 drop sage essential oil)
1 tsp. dried thyme (or 1 drop thyme essential oil)

WHAT TO DO:

1. Preheat oven to 325 degrees.
2. Sauté the chopped sausage until browned on all sides then set aside.
3. In a large skillet, melt the butter then add in the sage and thyme oils by stirring them in with a toothpick.
4. Add the chopped mushrooms, onions and celery. Once softened, mix in the sausage. When well combined, add in the remaining ingredients and combine well. Add more seasoning or herbs if you prefer.
5. Place stuffing in a baking dish and cover. Bake for about 20 minutes then remove the lid. Brown the top for about 10 minutes and then it is ready!

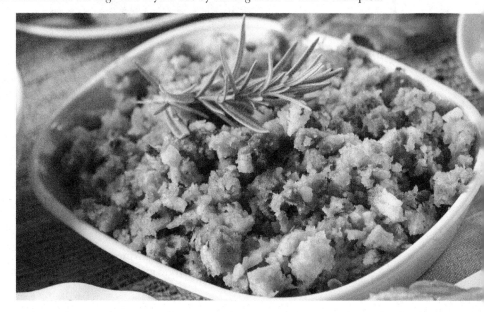

TWICE BAKED POTATOES WITH THYME, ONION AND GARLIC OIL

Serves 4

Baked potatoes are a great side dish for beef entrees and this recipe is infused with garlic and onion flavors that seep into the potatoes as they bake.

RECOMMENDED ESSENTIAL OILS:

1 drop of onion oil
1 drop of garlic oil
1 drop of thyme oil

WHAT YOU WILL NEED:

4-6 oz. medium potatoes (russet)
1 tsp. olive oil
11 tbsp. butter unsalted
2 leeks
2 tsp. fresh thyme (or 1 drop thyme essential oil)
4 oz. flavored cream cheese (chive and onion with reduced fat)
1/2 cup skim milk
Salt and pepper to taste
1 tbsp. chopped chives to top (optional)
Sour cream (optional)
2 garlic cloves (or 1 drop garlic essential oil)
1 drop onion essential oil

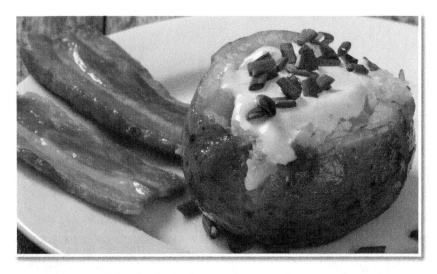

WHAT TO DO:

1. Preheat oven to 375 degrees and prepare a baking sheet.

2. Cover the potatoes in olive oil, salt, and line them up on the baking sheet.

3. Bake them for 1 hour to 1 1/2 hours. Once they are done, let them sit for 5-10 minutes.

4. In a sauce pan, melt the butter and add the leeks. Season them with salt and pepper and sauté them for about 5 minutes. About 10 minutes before the potatoes are finished you can start the next step.

5. Add in the minced garlic or garlic oil, fresh thyme or thyme oil, and onion oil. Saute for one minute.

6. Remove from heat and keep it ready for the potatoes.

7. When potatoes have cooled, slice each one open on one end and spoon out the insides of them into a bowl. Leave a thin layer of potato against the skin.

8. Mix the leek, butter, milk and cream cheese into the potatoes and blend well until there are just a few chunks.

9. Add the stuffing back into each potato skin. Now place them back into the oven and bake about 20 minutes. Top with sour cream and chives.

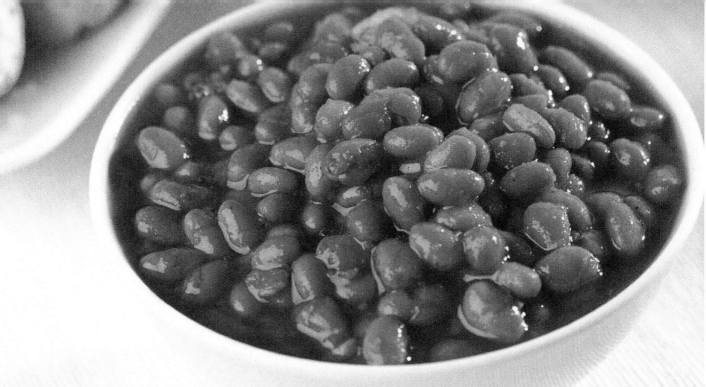

BAKED BEANS WITH ONION OIL

Serves 8

These rich baked beans have hints of molasses to make them sweet and mustard and vinegar to make them tangy.

RECOMMENDED ESSENTIAL OILS:

1 drop of onion oil

WHAT YOU WILL NEED:

4 oz. bacon (cooked and sliced)
1 onion, diced (or 1 drop onion essential oil)
Salt and pepper to taste
1 lb. dried navy beans (soak overnight and drain)
1/2 cup molasses
1/4 cup ketchup
1 tbsp. dry mustard
2 tbsp. cider vinegar

WHAT TO DO:

1. Preheat oven to 300 degrees.
2. In a Dutch oven, fry the bacon, then remove. Add the onion and cook in the grease, adding salt and pepper.
3. Next, add the beans, molasses, ketchup, water, mustard and onion oil. Stir well and heat to boiling.

4. Cover the pot and place in the oven. The liquid should reduce in half after about 2 and half hours.
5. Remove cover and stir. Place back in the oven for about an hour and a half longer.
6. Finally, stir in the vinegar, mix well and serve.

Chapter 16
Main Dishes

HAM AND CHEESE QUICHE WITH NUTMEG OIL

Serves 9

This is a cheesy blend of mozzarella and cheddar cheeses mixed with whisked creamy eggs all in a delicious pie crust.

RECOMMENDED ESSENTIAL OILS:

1 drop of nutmeg oil

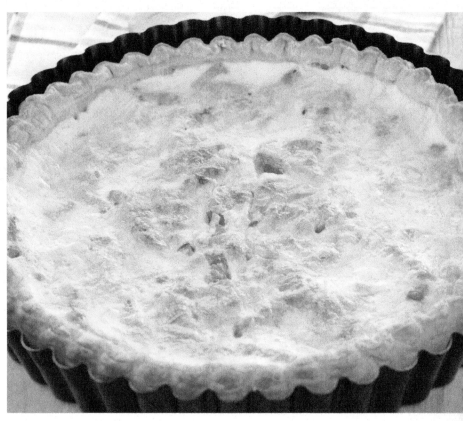

WHAT YOU WILL NEED:

4 large eggs

2 cups half and half cream

Pinch of salt

1/4 tsp. white pepper

4 oz. shredded cheddar cheese

2 oz. mozzarella cheese, shredded

1 9-inch pie shell (unbaked)

6 oz. chopped ham (optional)

1 tsp. ground nutmeg (or 1 drop nutmeg essential oil)

WHAT TO DO:

1. Preheat oven to 425 degrees.

2. In a mixing bowl, combine the eggs, cream, salt, pepper and nutmeg. If you are using ham (optional), add it in at this point. Whisk well.

3. Sprinkle a little ground nutmeg into the mixture or stir in nutmeg oil using the toothpick method. Set aside.

4. Sprinkle cheese on the pie crust, mixing the cheddar and mozzarella together.

5. Pour the egg mixture on top.

6. Bake for 15 minutes, then reduce heat to 350 degrees and continue baking for 20 more minutes. Check to see if the eggs are set and the crust is brown.

7. Let it cool for about 5 minutes before slicing and serving.

BACON, LETTUCE AND TOMATO SANDWICH WITH BASIL OIL

Serves 4

Enjoy this flavorful and indulgent sandwich with creamy mayonnaise infused with basil, succulent bacon, juicy tomato and a delicious new addition: the fried green tomato.

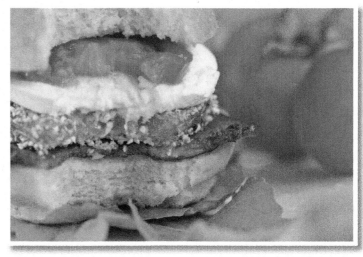

RECOMMENDED ESSENTIAL OILS:

2 drops of basil oil

WHAT YOU WILL NEED:

FOR THE MAYONNAISE:

1/4 fresh basil leaves (or 2 drops basil essential oil)

1/2 cup mayonnaise

1 tbsp. lemon juice (fresh squeezed)

Salt and pepper to taste

FOR THE TOMATOES:

2 green tomatoes, sliced

1/2 cup all-purpose flour

1/2 cup breadcrumbs

1 large egg

1 tbsp. milk

Olive oil as needed

Salt and pepper to taste

FOR THE SANDWICH:

4 rounds Port Madison goat cheese

1 large red tomato sliced

4 slices bacon

8 pieces bread or buns

WHAT TO DO:

1. For the mayonnaise, combine the basil leaves, mayonnaise, lemon juice and mustard together in a food processor and pulse until well combined.

2. Add salt and pepper to taste. You can enhance the flavor of the mayo with a few drops of basil oil. Start by using a toothpick dipped in the basil oil and stir it in. Depending on how strong the flavor is for your tastes, add more oil using the toothpick or a dropper. Stir well and set aside in the refrigerator.

3. To prepare the sandwiches, add the bacon slices to a large skillet and fry until browned on both sides. Once browned, remove and place on a lined paper towel dish to absorb excess grease.

4. Lay two slices of bread on each of four plates. Add the basil mayonnaise to the bread slices. Place one slice of bacon, folded in half, on each bread piece.

5. Next, add one round of goat cheese and slice of red tomato on each sandwich.

6. For the fried tomatoes, prepare a plate with a paper towel. Wash and slice each green tomato so that it is a half inch thick. Sprinkle with salt and pepper.

7. Prepare a small bowl by filling it with flour. In another bowl, add egg and milk whisked together, and in a third bowl, add the breadcrumbs.

8. Heat a large frying pan over medium to high heat and add about 1/2 inch of olive oil. Take each tomato slice and cover it in flour, then egg and milk and then breadcrumbs. Fry each coated tomato in the frying pan for about 3 minutes per side. Then transfer to the paper towel on the plate to soak up the extra oil. Once they have cooled down, place one on each sandwich. Enjoy!

RED PEPPER HUMMUS CHICKEN WRAP WITH BASIL OIL

Serves 4

Red pepper hummus adds just the right amount of flavor and texture to these veggie and chicken wraps to make for a great light lunch.

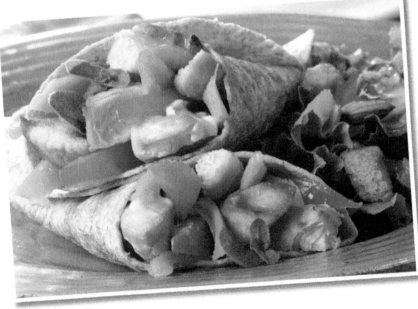

RECOMMENDED ESSENTIAL OILS:

2 drops of basil oil

WHAT YOU WILL NEED:

12 oz. sliced chicken breasts (cooked)
4 flour tortillas
1/2 cup red pepper hummus
1/2 cup carrots, shredded
1/2 sliced cucumber
2 tomatoes sliced and seeds removed
1 avocado, sliced
4 tbsp. fresh basil leaves (or 2 drops basil essential oil)
Salt and pepper to taste

WHAT TO DO:

1. Add 1 to 2 drops of basil oil into the hummus and blend well.
2. Lay out the tortillas and spread hummus on each one.
3. Add the veggies and chicken, season with salt and pepper, roll up and serve.

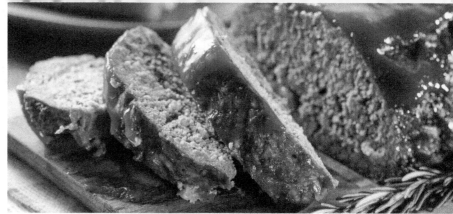

MEATLOAF WITH BLACK PEPPER, THYME AND CUMIN OIL

Serves 6-8

This meatloaf should be illegal it is so darn good! The glaze along with the vegetables baked in make it moist and flavorful.

RECOMMENDED ESSENTIAL OILS:

1 drop of black pepper oil
1 drop of thyme oil
1 drop of cumin oil

WHAT YOU WILL NEED:

6 oz. garlic-flavored croutons
1/2 tsp. cayenne pepper
1 tsp. chili powder
1/2 yellow onion, chopped
1 carrot, peeled and broken
3 cloves of garlic
1/2 bell pepper
18 oz. ground chuck
18 oz. ground sirloin
1 1/2 tsp. salt
1 large egg
½ tsp. ground black pepper (or 1 drop black pepper essential oil)
1 tsp. dried thyme (or 1 drop thyme essential oil)

FOR THE SAUCE:

1/2 cup ketchup
1 tsp. ground cumin (or 1 drop cumin essential oil)
Dash Worcestershire sauce
Dash hot sauce
1 tbsp. honey

WHAT TO DO:

1. Preheat oven to 325 degrees and line a baking sheet with parchment paper.

2. Combine the croutons, cayenne, and chili powder in a food processor and pulse.

3. Pour the mixture into a mixing bowl and process the chopped onion, carrot, pepper and garlic in the food processor until finely processed. Pour into crouton mix.

4. Add beef and salt. Stir well.

5. In a small bowl, whisk an egg. Add black pepper oil and thyme oil using the toothpick method. Mix well, then add that into the mixing bowl with the other ingredients. Combine well.

6. Once thoroughly mixed, place into a loaf pan 10 inches long. Turn the meatloaf onto the parchment paper and place it in the oven.

7. Prepare the glaze by combining all the sauce ingredients. Brush it onto the meatloaf after about 10 minutes of cooking.

8. Cook meatloaf for about 90 minutes, and check that the internal temperature is 155 degrees. Then it is ready!

SHRIMP SCAMPI AND LINGUINE WITH PARSLEY AND LEMON OIL

Serves 4-6

The shrimp, shallots and garlic absorb the butter, lemon and parsley flavors to bring life to this pasta dish.

RECOMMENDED ESSENTIAL OILS:

1 drop of parsley oil

3 drops of lemon oil

WHAT YOU NEED:

1 lb. linguini

4 tbsp. butter

4 tbsp. extra virgin olive oil

1 large shallot, finely diced

5 cloves of garlic, sliced

1 lb. shrimp, large (peeled and deveined, tail on)

Salt and pepper to taste

1/2 cup dry white wine

1 lemon for juice (or 3 drops lemon essential oil)

1/4 cup fresh parsley leaves, finely chopped (or 1 drop parsley essential oil)

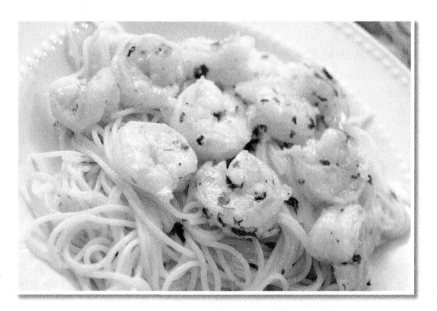

WHAT TO DO:

1. Bring a large pot of water to a boil and add a tablespoon of salt.

2. Drop the linguine noodles in. Allow them to boil for about 7 minutes, then drain. You want them cooked al dente. Save about 1 cup of the water.

3. In a large skillet, melt 2 tbsp. of butter and olive oil on medium heat.

4. Add in the garlic and shallot and allow them to soften up and turn translucent. Sprinkle salt and pepper on the shrimp and add them to the skillet and allow them to lose their translucency.

5. Pour in the wine, squeeze the juice from the lemon, and add the cup of water from earlier, along with the remaining butter and oil. Add the lemon and parsley essential oils. Bring to a boil.

6. Sprinkle in the chopped parsley leaves, the noodles and add the shrimp. Stir to combine then it is ready to serve.

FOIL-COOKED HERB SALMON WITH LEMON, PARSLEY AND BASIL OIL

Serves 2

The flavors of basil, lemon, garlic and parsley bubble and marinate together while absorbing into this salmon dish.

RECOMMENDED ESSENTIAL OILS:

3 drops of lemon oil

1 drop of parsley oil

1 drop of basil oil

WHAT YOU NEED:

2 cloves of garlic, minced

6 tbsp. olive oil

1 tsp. salt

1 tsp. ground black pepper

2-6 oz. salmon fillets

Fresh parsley, chopped

1 tbsp. lemon juice (or 3 drops lemon essential oil)

1 tbsp. fresh parsley, chopped (or 1 drop parsley essential oil)

1 tsp. dried basil (or 1 drop basil essential oil)

WHAT TO DO:

1. In a bowl, add the minced garlic, olive oil, salt, pepper, lemon juice, parsley, and dried basil, and/or their respective oils using the toothpick method. Mix well.

2. In a baking dish, lay out fillets in the oil mixture and let marinate in the fridge for about an hour.

3. Preheat oven to 375 degrees. Remove the fillets out of the fridge. Wrap each fillet in foil with some of the marinade and seal them. Place them in the dish and bake for about 40 minutes.

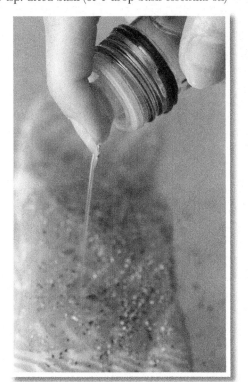

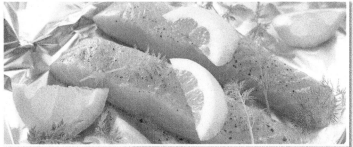

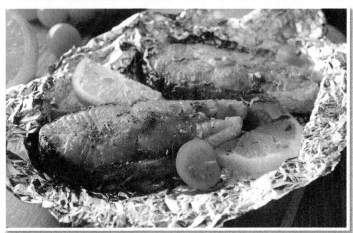

FAJITAS WITH LIME AND CILANTRO OIL

Serves 4-6

Enjoy blackened bell peppers and chicken slathered with guacamole, sour cream and salsa wrapped in a warm tortilla and infused with lime and cilantro.

RECOMMENDED ESSENTIAL OILS:

1 drop of coriander oil
2 drops of lime oil

WHAT YOU WILL NEED:

2 cloves garlic, minced
1/2 tsp. powdered chili
1/2 tsp. ground coriander
1/2 tsp. cumin
3 tbsp. olive oil
1 lb. chicken breasts
Salt and pepper to taste
1 red bell pepper, sliced
1 red onion, sliced
8 6-inch tortillas
Guacamole
Sour Cream
Salsa
1/3 cup fresh cilantro (and 1 drop coriander essential oil)
1 juice of lime (or 2 drops lime essential oil)

WHAT TO DO:

1. To prepare the marinade for the chicken, mix 2 tablespoons of olive oil with cilantro oil, garlic, chili powder, coriander, cumin and lime oil. Mix well.

2. Add the chicken and bell peppers into the marinade. Let them soak in the mixture for 2 hours in the fridge.

3. When you are ready to grill, heat up a grilling pan and add the chicken pieces.

4. Add salt and pepper. Grill until darkened on one side, then flip and darken the other side. Once thoroughly cooked, remove the chicken and add the bell peppers. Allow them to blacken in spots.

5. Warm up the tortillas on a clean surface. Be sure to warm both sides then wrap them in a clean dish towel.

6. Slice the chicken and mix it with the bell peppers. Fill each warm tortilla with chicken, peppers and guacamole, sour cream and/or salsa. Self-serve stations are nice for these fajitas.

POT ROAST WITH MARJORAM, THYME AND OREGANO OIL

Serves 6

What's for dinner? Here's a melt-in-your-mouth pot roast infused with thyme and oregano to enjoy.

RECOMMENDED ESSENTIAL OILS:

1 drop of oregano oil
1 drop of thyme oil
1 drop of marjoram oil

WHAT YOU WILL NEED:

2 lbs. boneless chuck roast (beef)
9 red potatoes (small)
1 ½ cups carrots, chopped
1 onion, quartered
1 tsp. beef bouillon granules
1/4 tsp. pepper
1/2 tsp. salt
1/2 tsp. garlic powder
1/2 cup water
1 tsp. dried oregano (or 1 drop oregano essential oil)
1 tsp. dried thyme (or 1 drop thyme essential oil)
1 tsp. dried marjoram (or 1 drop marjoram essential oil)

WHAT TO DO:

1. Preheat oven to 350 degrees. In a 9-inch x 13-inch baking dish, add the roast and all the chopped vegetables.

2. Sprinkle the bouillon salt and garlic powder on the roast and vegetables.

3. For the marjoram, thyme and oregano: if you are using the actual herbs sprinkle them on the roast and vegetables. If you are using the oils, dip a toothpick into the oil and swirl it in the 1/2 cup of water, then pour the water on top of the roast.

4. Wrap a pan in a layer of foil and bake for 2 1/2 hours. Serve immediately with warm bread.

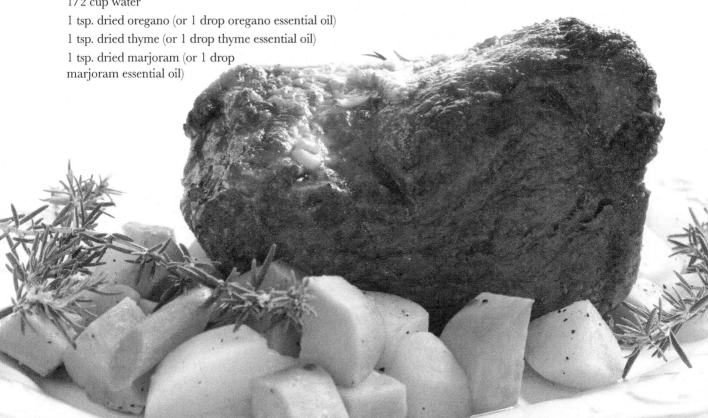

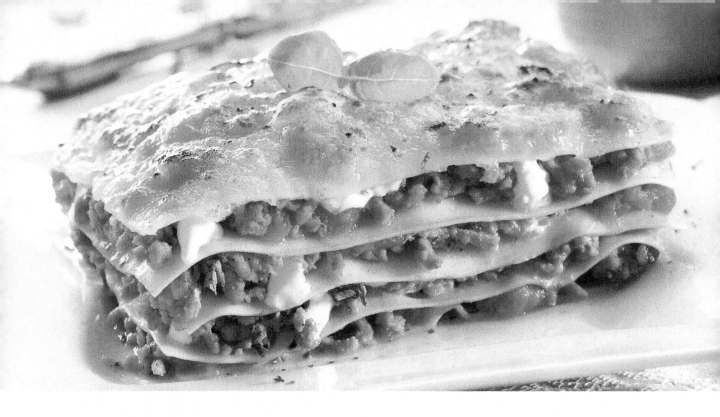

LASAGNA WITH BASIL AND FENNEL OIL

Serves 12

Make a homemade lasagna, piled high with delicious cheeses, tomatoes, sweet Italian sausages and beef. Don't forget the infusion of Italian spices!

RECOMMENDED ESSENTIAL OILS:

1 drop of basil oil
1 drop of fennel oil

WHAT YOU WILL NEED:

1 lb. Italian sausage (sweet)
3/4 lb. ground beef
1/2 cup onions, minced
2 crushed cloves of garlic
28 oz. canned tomatoes
1/2 cup water
2 tbsp. granulated sugar
1 tsp. Italian seasoning
1 tbsp. salt

1/4 tsp. black pepper
4 tbsp. parsley
12 lasagna noodles
16 oz. ricotta cheese
1 large egg
1/2 tsp. salt
3/4 lb. mozzarella cheese, sliced
3/4 cup parmesan cheese, grated
1 ½ tsp. dried basil (or 1 drop basil essential oil)
½ tsp. fennel seeds (or 1 drop fennel essential oil)

1. Preheat oven to 375 degrees. Combine the beef, sausage, onions, and garlic together in a stock pot. Cook over medium heat. Keep stirring and brown all the meat thoroughly.

2. Stir in the tomato paste, sauce and crushed tomatoes. Blend well.

3. Add in water, sugar, basil oil or leaves, fennel oil or seeds, Italian seasonings, 2 tablespoons of parsley, salt and pepper. Stir well then lower heat to simmer.

4. Cover and cook for about an hour and a half.

5. In another large pot, add water and a pinch of salt and bring to a boil. Add in lasagna noodles and boil for 8 minutes so that they are softened but still a little stiff. When finished, drain the water and rinse the noodles. Set them aside.

6. In another bowl, add ricotta cheese in with the remaining parsley, 1/2 teaspoon of sea salt and a whisked egg.

7. For the lasagna, prepare a 9 inch by 13 inch baking dish for filling. Pour the meat sauce in the bottom, lay 6 noodles to cover the meat sauce, then cover the noodles with a ricotta cheese and egg layer.

8. Next, add a layer of mozzarella cheese slices. After that is another meat sauce layer covered in 1/4 of the parmesan cheese. Repeat again meat sauce, noodles, ricotta cheese, mozzarella, meat sauce and parmesan. The top layer should be parmesan and mozzarella cheese.

9. Cover the dish with foil. Be sure the foil doesn't stick to the cheese. Bake for 50 minutes. Cover the lasagna for the first 25 minutes, then remove the foil for the last 25 minutes.

Tip:

Give your pizza, ravioli, or lasagna pizzazz like it's from the ole country by adding oregano, marjoram, thyme, or basil to your tomato sauce. Toothpick method is preferred.

Chapter 17
Breads

APPLE AND CINNAMON MUFFINS WITH CINNAMON OIL

Serves 12

Try this warm and crumbly muffin filled with flavors of apples and cinnamon. If you are a fan of walnuts or pecans, add them into the topping to get an extra crunch.

RECOMMENDED ESSENTIAL OILS:

1 drop of cinnamon oil

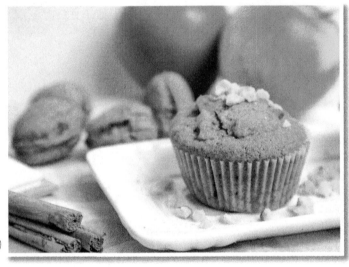

WHAT YOU WILL NEED:

1 1/2 cup all-purpose flour

1/3 cup granulated sugar

2 tsp. baking powder

1/2 tsp. salt

1 large egg

1/2 cup milk

1 apple (remove skin, core and then chop)

4 tbsp. melted butter

1/3 cup chopped walnuts or pecans (optional)

1/4 cup brown sugar (packed)

1/2 tsp. ground cinnamon (or 1 drop cinnamon essential oil)

1 tsp. honey

WHAT TO DO:

1. Preheat oven to 375 degrees. Grease a muffin baking tray or add in paper liners.

2. In a large bowl, mix the dry ingredients: flour, sugar, 1/2 teaspoon of ground cinnamon, salt and baking powder.

3. In another bowl, mix up the wet ingredients. Start with the egg and whisk it with the milk. Then add in the chopped apple and butter. Once well combined, mix the wet ingredients into the dry. Blend well.

4. Once all ingredients are well incorporated, divide them between 12 muffin cups.

5. Prepare the topping by mixing 1 teaspoon of honey with a drop of cinnamon oil (if you have the essential oil) in a bowl.

6. Add the brown sugar and mix well. If you are going to use nuts, chop them finely and then mix them into the sugar mixture well.

7. Divide this mixture between the muffin cups evenly.

8. Bake for 15 minutes. They should be a nice toasty brown on their tops. Remove from the pan and let cool. Serve them warm or keep them in an airtight container for later.

SPICED ZUCCHINI BREAD WITH VANILLA AND CINNAMON OIL

Makes 2 loaves

This bread is speckled with shredded zucchini and has hints of vanilla and cinnamon throughout. It is easy to make and sure to fill your kitchen with a great smell.

RECOMMENDED ESSENTIAL OILS:

1 drop of vanilla oil
1-2 drops of cinnamon oil

WHAT YOU WILL NEED:

2 cups zucchini (shredded)
2 tsp. ground cinnamon (or 1-2 drops cinnamon essential oil)
3 large eggs
1 1/3 cups sugar
1/2 cup vegetable oil
1/2 cup applesauce
2 1/2 cups all-purpose flour
1/4 tsp. baking powder
2 tsp. baking soda
1 tsp. salt
1 3/4 cups walnuts chopped (optional)
2 tsp. pure vanilla extract (and 1 drop vanilla essential oil)

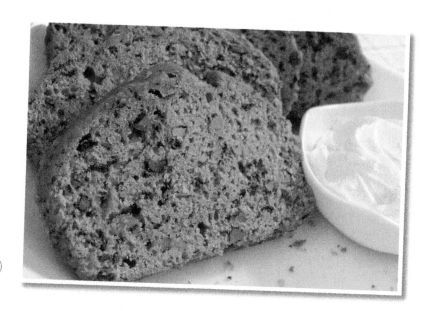

WHAT TO DO:

1. Preheat oven to 350 degrees. Prepare two 8 1/2 by 4 1/2 inch loaf pans by greasing and flouring them.

2. Shred the zucchini and place it into a strainer. Squeeze the liquid out by pressing down on the zucchini.

3. In a separate bowl, combine the sugar, eggs, oil and applesauce together and mix well.

4. Mix in the cinnamon and vanilla oils by using a toothpick. Dip the toothpick in each oil and then swirl it into the mixture.

5. Add in the flour, baking soda, cinnamon, baking powder, salt and chopped walnuts, if desired.

6. Divide the mix between the two loaf pans and bake them for 50 minutes. Test if they're done by inserting a toothpick into the middle and looking for no crumbs to stick to it. Once finished, remove them from the oven and allow them to cool.

7. To serve, slice and serve warm with butter.

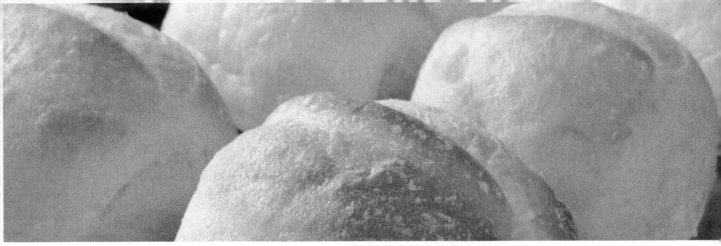

HERB DINNER ROLLS WITH THYME AND ROSEMARY OIL

Serves 12 (24 rolls)

Perfect rolls for a variety of occasions.

RECOMMENDED ESSENTIAL OILS:

1 drop of rosemary oil

1 drop of thyme oil

WHAT YOU WILL NEED:

1 1/2 tsp. salt

5 cups bread flour

1 cup milk

1/4 cup butter

1/3 cup sugar

2 packages of yeast (dry)

2 large eggs

2 tbsp. butter (melted)

1 tbsp. fresh rosemary (or 1 drop rosemary essential oil)

1 tbsp. fresh thyme (or 1 drop thyme essential oil)

WHAT TO DO:

1. In a large bowl, combine 1 1/2 cups of bread flour and salt. If you are using fresh herbs, add them into the bread flour now.

2. In a small sauce pan, heat up the milk, sugar and butter over low heat. If you are using essential oil, use a toothpick to stir in the rosemary and thyme oils.

3. Once the milk mixture is warm, add the yeast. It should become foamy and brown. Next, gradually mix the yeast mixture into the bread flour bowl.

4. Beat rapidly for about 2 minutes. Once smooth, beat in an egg and 1/2 cup of bread flour. Keep beating it for 2 more minutes. You want a soft dough. Keep adding in flour until the dough becomes soft. You can add more as you are kneading the dough.

5. The average amount of bread flour is 5 cups, but it may vary due to humidity levels. Once your dough is soft, knead it on a floured surface for about 10 minutes.

6. Grease a mixing bowl. Roll the dough into a ball and place it in the bowl. Cover the bowl and place it in a warm, dark place to rise for about an hour.

7. Preheat the oven to 400 degrees.

8. Punch the dough down and divide it into two. Cover one half. Break the other half into 12 rolls and place them on a baking sheet about 2 inches apart. Cover them and place them in a warm, dark place for about a half an hour to rise again. As those are rising, work on the other half of dough and do the same.

9. Once the rolls have doubled in size, spread melted butter on the top and bake them for about 10 minutes. They should be golden brown. Serve with your dinner.

CINNAMON RAISIN ROLLS WITH CINNAMON AND VANILLA OIL

Serves 6 (12 rolls)

What is better to wake up to than the smell of baking cinnamon rolls and fresh coffee? Enjoy these sweet and gooey breakfast treats.

RECOMMENDED ESSENTIAL OILS:

2 drops of cinnamon oil
1 drop of vanilla oil

WHAT YOU NEED:

FOR THE BREAD:

1/4 oz. yeast
1/2 cup warm water
1/2 cup hot milk
1/4 cup granulated sugar
1/3 cup butter
1 tsp. salt
1 large egg
3 1/2 cups flour

FOR THE FILLING:

2 tsp. ground cinnamon (or 2 drops cinnamon essential oil)
1/2 cup melted butter
3/4 cup sugar
3/4 cup raisins (optional)

FOR THE GLAZE:

4 tbsp. butter
2 cups powdered sugar
1 tsp. vanilla extract (or 1 drop vanilla essential oil)
4 tbsp. hot water

WHAT TO DO:

1. First you will need to make the bread for the rolls from scratch so it will take a little time.

2. In a small bowl, add the warm water and the yeast and allow it to dissolve.

3. In a large bowl, add the milk, sugar, egg, drops of cinnamon and melted butter and mix well.

4. Stir in 2 cups of flour until smooth. Once smooth, you will pour in the water and yeast combination and mix in the other cup and a half of flour.

5. Flour a wooden surface and knead the mixture for about 10 minutes.

6. Grease a bowl and then place the dough into it. Cover it with a greased piece of plastic and then a damp towel. Allow it to sit in a draft-free area for about an hour and a half. It will double in size. After that time has passed, flour the surface again. Then roll out the dough and make a rectangle that is about 15 inches by 9 inches.

7. To prepare the filling, cover the rectangle in melted butter. Then, in a small bowl mix the cinnamon and sugar and sprinkle it all over the dough. Next, spread the raisins out.

8. On the long side of the rectangle, begin to roll it up. Once it is rolled seal it as best as you can. Next, slice it into 12 rolls.

9. Prepare a baking pan by covering the base with butter and sugar. Then place the rolls on the pan and cover again with oiled plastic and let sit for about an hour. They will double in size again.

10. Preheat oven to 350 degrees. When the rolls have finished rising, place them into the oven for about 25-30 minutes. They will smell amazing as they cook and should be lightly browned on the top.

11. While those are baking, mix the delicious frosting. In a bowl, combine the butter, sugar and vanilla.

12. Add hot water gradually until you have your desired consistency.

13. When the rolls are finished baking and have cooled a little bit, spread the frosting and serve!

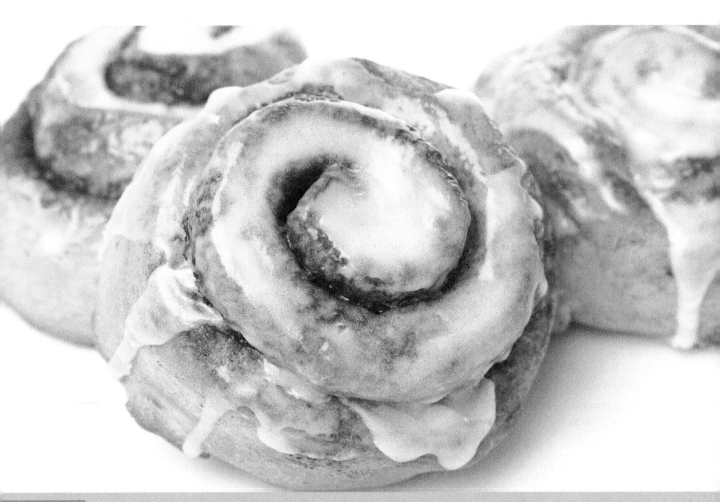

Chapter 18
Desserts

CHOCOLATE CHIP COOKIES WITH PEPPERMINT OIL

Makes 24-30 cookies

These flat, crispy cookies are crunchy bite-sized treats that make a great snack anytime!

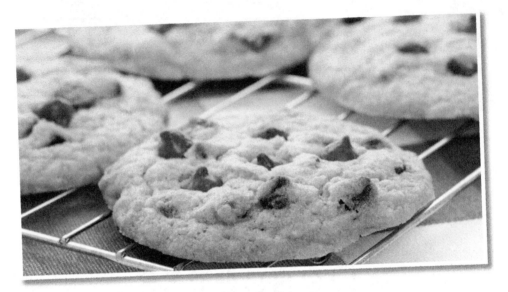

RECOMMENDED ESSENTIAL OILS:

1-3 drops of peppermint oil

WHAT YOU WILL NEED:

1/4 lb. butter, unsalted
1 cup brown sugar
1/2 cup sugar
2 eggs
1 tsp. vanilla extract
1-3 drops peppermint essential oil
1 1/2 cups flour
1/2 tsp. salt
1/2 tsp. baking soda
1 cup chocolate chips

WHAT TO DO:

1. Preheat oven to 375 degrees. Spray baking sheet with non-stick cooking spray.

2. In a large bowl, sift together all of the dry ingredients. In another bowl, cream butter, adding sugar gradually and beat until smooth.

3. Add in eggs, vanilla extract and peppermint essential oil.

4. Slowly add dry ingredients into the wet mixture and stir until well blended. Fold in chocolate chips.

5. Drop a tablespoon of cookie dough per cookie onto baking sheet, leaving 2 inches between them to allow room for spreading.

6. Bake until golden brown, approximately 8-10 minutes. Remove cookies immediately from cookie sheet and allow to cool.

Tip:
Spice up ginger snap cookies with ginger, cinnamon, clove bud, or nutmeg. Add to cookie dough using the toothpick method.

PUMPKIN AND CREAM CHEESE SWIRL LOAF WITH GINGER AND NUTMEG OIL

Serves 10

Bite into a slice of this swirled pumpkin bread and get a taste of the sweet filling that perfectly complements the pumpkin bread.

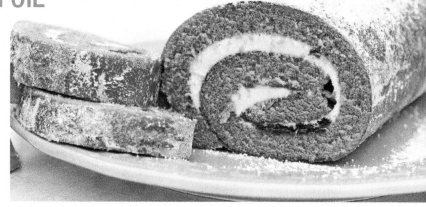

RECOMMENDED ESSENTIAL OILS:

1 drop of cinnamon oil

1 drop of ginger oil

1 drop of nutmeg oil

WHAT YOU WILL NEED:

3 eggs

1 cup granulated sugar

2/3 cup pumpkin

1 tsp. lemon juice

3/4 cup flour

1 tsp. baking powder

1/2 tsp. salt

2 tsp. ground cinnamon (or 1 drop cinnamon essential oil)

1 tsp. ground ginger (or 1 drop ginger essential oil)

1/2 tsp. ground nutmeg (or 1 drop nutmeg essential oil)

FOR THE CREAM FILLING:

8 oz. cream cheese

4 tbsp. butter

1 cup powdered sugar

1/2 tsp. vanilla extract

WHAT TO DO:

1. Preheat oven to 350 degrees. Grease and line a 10-inch by 15-inch shallow pan with wax paper.

2. In a bowl, mix the eggs and sugar together until smooth, preferably with an electric mixer.

3. Add in the lemon juice and pumpkin.

4. In another bowl, mix the dry ingredients including the flour, baking powder and salt. If using dry spices add them into the dry bowl.

5. If adding essential oils using the toothpick method, stir them into the wet ingredients. Then, add the wet ingredients into the dry ingredients and mix until smooth.

6. Pour the batter into the pan and spread it evenly. Bake 15 minutes, then let it cool off for about 15 minutes.

7. Spread powdered sugar on a tea towel and place the cake on it. Roll up the cake from one of the 10-inch sides. Set that to the side and whip up the filling.

8. Mix together all filling ingredients until smooth. Then roll the cake back out and spread the filling over the surface of the cake.

9. Get a piece of plastic ready that you can wrap the roll in. Roll the cake up and wrap it. Place it in the fridge for an hour then it will be ready to slice and enjoy.

ORANGE BUNDT CAKE AND ORANGE FROSTING WITH ORANGE AND LEMON OIL

Serves 6-8

This light and airy bundt cake will fill your mouth with an orange zest when you take your first bite.

RECOMMENDED ESSENTIAL OILS:

2 drops of orange oil

1 drop of lemon oil

WHAT YOU WILL NEED:

1/2 cup soft butter

1 cup granulated sugar

2 large eggs

1/2 tsp. vanilla extract

1/4 tsp. almond extract

1 1/2 cups flour

1 1/2 tsp. baking powder

1/2 cup milk

FOR THE FROSTING:

1 cup powdered sugar

4 tsp. orange juice

1 1/2 tsp. orange zest (or 1 drop orange essential oil)

1/2 tsp. lemon extract (or 1 drop lemon essential oil)

WHAT TO DO:

1. In a mixing bowl, combine the butter and sugar until well combined. Beat the eggs as you stir them in, along with the vanilla and almond extract.

2. In another bowl, mix the flour and baking powder together. Stir it into the sugar mixture while taking turns stirring in the milk.

3. Preheat oven to 350 degrees.

4. Pour the batter into a floured fluted tube pan and bake for 45 minutes. You can insert a toothpick to make sure it is done throughout.

5. Once done, remove the cake from the pan and let it cool.

6. For the frosting, add the sugar and orange juice into a bowl. Stir in one drop of orange essential oil and one drop of lemon essential oil. Once the cake has cooled, spoon it over the top. Sprinkle orange or lemon zest on top.

Tip:

Add zest to your sponge or bundt cake by swirling a drop of lemon, orange, or tangerine essential oil into the cake batter.

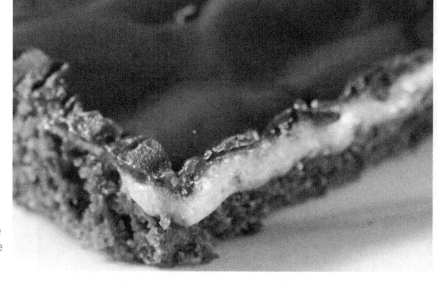

MINT CHOCOLATE CHEESECAKE BROWNIES WITH PEPPERMINT OIL

Serves 24

Try these delicious chocolate fudge brownies filled with a cream cheese minty layer.

RECOMMENDED ESSENTIAL OILS:

1 drop of peppermint oil

WHAT YOU WILL NEED:

1/2 cup salted butter

8 oz. chocolate semi-sweet, chopped

1 1/4 cups granulated sugar

3 eggs

1 tsp. vanilla extract

3/4 cup flour

1/4 tsp. salt

FOR THE MINT LAYER:

8 oz. softened cream cheese

1/4 cup granulated sugar

1 egg yolk

2 drops of green food coloring

2/3 cup mini chocalote chips

1/4 tsp. peppermint extract (or 1 drop peppermint essential oil)

WHAT TO DO:

1. Preheat oven to 350 degrees. Prepare a 13-inch x 9-inch baking dish with non-stick cooking spray.

2. Set out the cream cheese so it can soften.

3. In a medium saucepan, add the butter and chocolate from the brownie ingredients.

4. As the chocolate melts, stir and pay careful attention so it doesn't burn.

5. Cool the mixture back to room temperature, then stir in the eggs one by one. Once smooth, whisk in the vanilla. Add in the salt and flour. Stir well.

6. Spread 3/4 of the batter into the baking pan.

7. For the mint layer in a separate bowl, add the cream cheese, sugar, egg yolk, food coloring and peppermint oil. Beat until smooth, then stir in the mini chocolates gently.

8. Pour the mint layer over the brownie layer.

9. Top with the last layer of the brownie mix. Bake for about 30 minutes and check with a toothpick to see if anything sticks when inserted into the center of the brownies. If not, they are done! Let cool, then cut into squares.

 Tip:

If you are a Girl Scout thin mint cookie lover, try adding peppermint or spearmint essential oil to your recipes for chocolate cookies, brownies, or chocolate frosting mixes.

PUMPKIN PIE WITH CLOVE, NUTMEG AND GINGER OIL

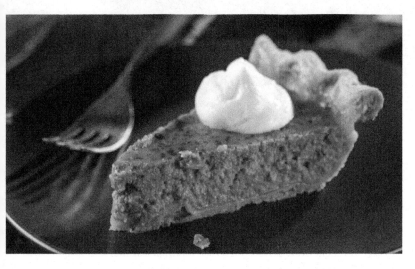

Serves 8

With a crumbly crust, this melt-in-your-mouth cinnamon pumpkin pie is complete with a dollop of whip cream.

RECOMMENDED ESSENTIAL OILS:

1 drop of clove oil
1 drop of nutmeg oil
1 drop of ginger oil

WHAT YOU WILL NEED:

2 cups pumpkin
1 1/2 cups heavy cream
1/2 cup dark brown sugar
1/3 cup granulated sugar
1/2 tsp. salt
2 eggs
1 egg yolk
2 tsp. cinnamon
1 tsp. ground ginger (or 1 drop ginger essential oil)
1/4 tsp. ground cardamom
1 cooked pie crust
1/4 tsp. ground nutmeg (plus, 1 drop nutmeg essential oil)
1/4 tsp. ground cloves (plus, 1 drop clove essential oil)

WHAT TO DO:

1. Preheat oven to 425 degrees.
2. In a mixing bowl, combine the sugar and salt. Add the eggs gradually.
3. Next, add in the pumpkin and cream. Mix until thoroughly combined.
4. Then using a toothpick, add in the clove, nutmeg and ginger oils. Dip the toothpick in the oil and then stir it in the mix. Be careful to add it sparingly as the flavors can be strong.
5. Add in the remaining dry spices. When all mixed in, pour the pumpkin filling into the pie crust and bake for 15 minutes.
6. Lower oven temperature to 350 degrees and bake for 45 minutes.
7. Remove pie from oven and let cool for 2 hours. Serve slices topped with whipped cream.

 Tip:

When the holidays roll around, try spicing up your pumpkin pie or spice cake by adding nutmeg, cinnamon, clove bud, or ginger essential oil to your recipe.

LEMON CHEESECAKE WITH LEMON OIL

Serves 10

Light cheesecake infused with sweet lemon flavor makes a fresh dessert.

RECOMMENDED ESSENTIAL OILS:

8 drops of lemon oil

WHAT YOU WILL NEED:

6 oz. biscuits, baked

1/6 lb. melted butter

7 oz. cream cheese

9 oz. mascarpone

1 1/2 tbsp. yogurt

7 tbsp. powdered sugar

1 additional lemon for juice and peels

1 lemon zest (and 8 drops lemon essential oil)

WHAT TO DO:

1. Make the crust of this cake by placing baked biscuits in a Ziploc bag and crushing them all up.

2. In a bowl, add the melted butter and pour the biscuit crumbs into it. Mix thoroughly, then press into a pie dish. Place in the fridge.

3. In another bowl, mix the cream cheese, yogurt, mascarpone and sugar until nice and smooth.

4. Add in the drops of lemon oil, lemon juice and zest. Mix well and then pour into the biscuit crust.

5. Place in the fridge for 4 hours and then serve.

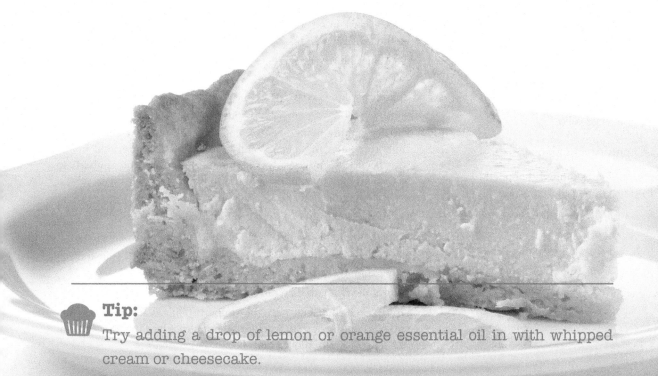

Tip:
Try adding a drop of lemon or orange essential oil in with whipped cream or cheesecake.

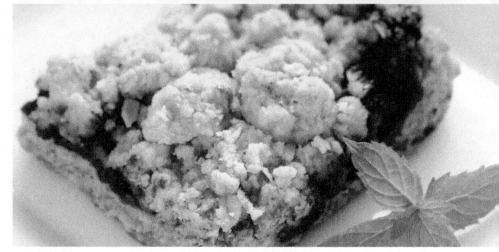

SHORTBREAD BARS AND RHUBARB WITH CARDAMOM OIL

Serves 18

Another delicious way to use rhubarb is in these rhubarb shortbread bars.

RECOMMENDED ESSENTIAL OILS:

1 drop of cardamom oil

WHAT YOU WILL NEED:

FOR THE CRUST:

1 cup flour

1 cup flour (light spelt)

1 tsp. baking powder

1 pinch salt

1 cup butter unsalted

1 cup sugar (cane)

2 egg yolks

FOR THE RHUBARB FILLING:

2 cups rhubarb, chopped

1/2 cup strawberries

1/3 cup sugar (cane)

1 tbsp. water

1 tsp. vanilla extract

2 tsp. ground cardamom (or 1 drop cardamom essential oil)

WHAT TO DO:

1. To make the dough, combine all of the dry ingredients in a bowl.
2. In another bowl, add the butter, yolks and sugar. Be sure to beat the wet mixture until fluffy.
3. If using cardamom oil, stir into the wet ingredients using the toothpick method. If using dry cardamom, add it into the dry ingredients.
4. Combine the dry ingredients into the wet to make a dough that is soft.
5. Split the dough into two balls, one slightly smaller than the other and wrap them in plastic. Freeze them for at least 45 minutes.
6. For the yummy filling, place a saucepan on low heat and add the rhubarb, water and sugar. While stirring the mixture, add in the strawberries. Gently stir for 15 minutes, allowing the rhubarb to soften and the sauce to thicken. If you prefer a thicker sauce, add in cornstarch as needed.
7. When it is done, remove from heat and add in vanilla.
8. Preheat oven to 350 degrees and grease a 10-inch spring form pan.
9. Remove the biggest dough ball out from the freezer and grate it using a cheese grater into the base of the pan.
10. Pour in the rhubarb filling to cover it.
11. Grate the second ball over the rhubarb filling. Pat it down gently and place in the oven to bake for 30 minutes. Once the top is golden brown, remove from oven and slice into bars.

ROSEMARY POUND CAKE AND FRUIT TOPPING WITH JUNIPER BERRY AND ROSEMARY OIL

Serves 8-9

Rosemary adds a new flavor this to pound cake which is then topped with a sweet fruit sauce.

RECOMMENDED ESSENTIAL OILS:

2 drops of juniper berry oil
2 drops of cinnamon oil
2 drops of rosemary oil

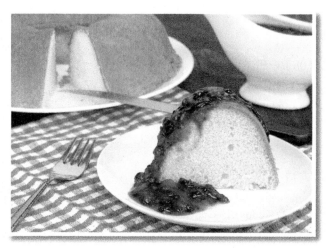

WHAT YOU WILL NEED:

2 cups mixed dehydrated fruits
1 tsp. peppercorns
1 cup port wine
1 2/3 cups granulated sugar
16 tbsp. butter (unsalted)
1 1/4 cups flour
1/4 tsp. baking powder
1/2 tsp. salt
3 large eggs
3 egg yolks
1/2 tsp. vanilla
8 juniper berries (and 1 drop juniper essential oil)
2 cinnamon sticks (and 2 drops cinnamon essential oil)
4 sprigs rosemary (or 1 drop rosemary essential oil)

WHAT TO DO:

1. Start by collecting all of your dried fruits and chopping them up into small pieces.

2. Next, add the juniper berries and/or juniper berry oil and peppercorns into a small saucepan and pour in the wine port and 2/3 cup of the sugar. Heat it over medium heat and stir.

3. Add in cinnamon sticks or cinnamon oil.

4. Finally, add in the chopped fruits and let them soak for about 5 minutes.

5. Remove the pan from the heat and let it cool for an hour.

6. Preheat oven to 350 degrees and grease three mini loaf pans. They should measure approximately 5 3/4-inch x 3 1/8-inch in size.

7. In another sauce pan, melt the butter and add 3 of the rosemary sprigs and/or rosemary oil. Cover with lid on and let it sit for 15 minutes.

Then remove the rosemary, if you used sprigs, by straining the liquid and reserving it in another bowl. Chop the leaves off the other rosemary sprigs and mix them with the flour, baking powder and salt. Mix well.

8. In another bowl, combine the whole eggs with the yolks and the vanilla rapidly until thoroughly whisked.

9. Beat in 1 cup of sugar until it thickens. Slowly stir in the dry ingredients gradually, while mixing on low speed. Then speed up the mixing to add in the rosemary butter. Beat until well-combined then pour it into the pans.

10. Bake the loaves for about 40 minutes until you see a dome shape. Be sure they are cooked throughout then invert them to cool. Once they have cooled, slice the loaves and serve them topped with the fruit mixture.

WHITE CHOCOLATE STRAWBERRY CAKE WITH ROSE OIL

Serves 10-12

This beautiful strawberry cake also has hints of rose baked into it.

RECOMMENDED ESSENTIAL OILS:

1 drop of rose oil

WHAT YOU WILL NEED:

FOR THE CAKE:

4 cups cake flour

2 tsp. baking powder

1 1/2 tsp. baking soda

1 tsp. salt

1 cup (2 sticks) unsalted butter, softened to room temperature

2 cups sugar

1 tbsp. pure vanilla extract

4 large eggs, at room temperature

2 cups buttermilk

1/2 cup white chocolate chunks

FOR THE FROSTING:

3 cups heavy whipping cream

1/4 cup powdered sugar

3 tbsp. rose water (or 1 drop rose essential oil)

2 tsp. pure vanilla extract

FOR THE FILLING:

1/2 cup finely chopped white chocolate chunks

1 1/2 cups sliced strawberries

Fresh rose petals or strawberries, for topping the cake

WHAT TO DO:

1. Place racks in the center and upper third of the oven and preheat oven to 350 degrees. Butter and flour two 9-inch round cake pans. This is a triple layer cake, so butter and flour three 9-inch cake pans if you have them.

2. In a large bowl, whisk together flour, baking powder, baking soda, and salt. Set aside.

3. In the bowl of an electric stand mixer fitted with a paddle attachment, beat butter and sugar at medium speed until pale and fluffy, about 3 to 4 minutes.

4. Add eggs one at a time, beating well and scraping down the bowl after each addition. Beat in vanilla extract.

5. Turn the mixer speed to low and add half of the dry ingredients. Add half of the buttermilk and beat until just combined. Add the remaining flour and buttermilk and beat until just combined. Remove the bowl from the stand mixer and finish incorporating the batter with a spatula. Scrape the bottom of the bowl to make sure there is no butter or flour hiding down there. Fold in the chocolate chips.

6. Divide the batter among the two cake pans, making sure that you save enough batter for the last cake to bake off. If you have three pans, divide the batter in three.

7. Spread batter evenly in each pan then rap each pan on the counter top to help the batter settle and eliminate any air bubbles.

8. Bake until bubbled and golden brown, about 20-25 minutes. Insert a toothpick into the center

of the cake. If it comes out dry with just a few crumbs, it's done! Cool cakes in the pan for 10 minutes before inverting onto a wire rack to cool completely. If you're baking off your last cake round, be sure to re-grease and flour the pan before adding the last of the cake batter.

9. To make the frosting, combine heavy cream, powdered sugar, and rose water or rose oil in the bowl of a stand mixer fitted with a whisk attachment. Beat on medium speed until soft peaks form. Once soft peaks form in the whipped cream, keep an eye on it. Continue beating just past the soft peak stage. You don't want to over-beat the whipped cream. It should hold its shape but still be smooth and spreadable. You can always beat the whipped cream into more shape, but you can't unwhip it to a smoother consistency once it's firm.

10. To assemble the cake, place three strips of parchment paper onto a cake plate or cake stand.

Place one cooled cake round atop the parchment paper. The paper will help keep the cake plate clean while you frost the cake.

11. Spread a generous amount of whipped cream atop the first layer. Arrange half of the sliced strawberries atop the whipped cream and sprinkle with half of the finely chopped white chocolate.

12. Place another cake layer atop the frosted layer. Top with more whipped cream, the remaining sliced strawberries, and sprinkle with the remaining white chocolate. Top with the last cake layer. Spread whipped cream across the top of the cake and smooth along the sides. Keep a tall glass of warm water nearby. Rinsing the knife clean will help smooth with whipped cream more easily.

13. To finish the cake, top with fresh rose petals in the center or strawberries as pictured.

14. Store cake in the fridge until ready to serve. To serve, remove a few of the petals and slice through the cake.

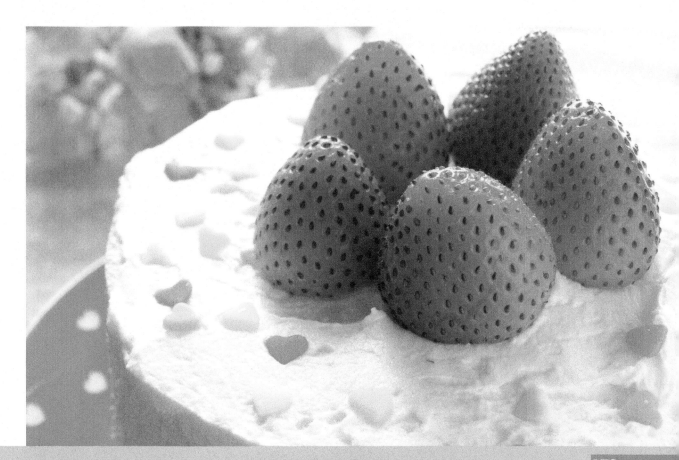

KEY LIME MOUSSE WITH LIME OIL

Serves 6

This is a cool refreshing treat of creamy chilled limes.

RECOMMENDED ESSENTIAL OILS:

1 drop of lime oil

WHAT YOU WILL NEED:

2/3 cup lime juice

2 tbsp. sugar

2 tsp. gelatin (unflavored)

Green food coloring (optional)

1 can condensed milk (sweet)

1 cup whipping cream

1 lime sliced

1 tbsp. lime peel, grated (or 1 drop lime essential oil)

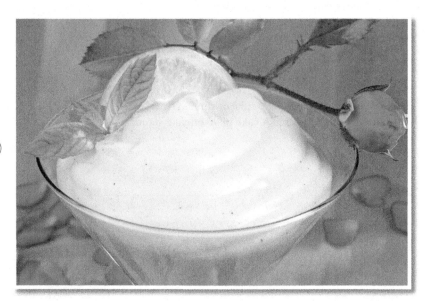

WHAT TO DO:

1. Start by mixing the lime juice, sugar and gelatin together in a sauce pan, heating over medium heat. Stir it so the gelatin dissolves.

2. Add in the lime zest or lime oil. If you are using food coloring, add it in and stir.

3. Remove from the heat and let it cool for about 5 minutes.

4. Add in milk and stir. Cover and place in the fridge for about 15 minutes. It should thicken.

5. Add the whip cream in with the other ingredients. Serve in glasses garnished with lime slices.

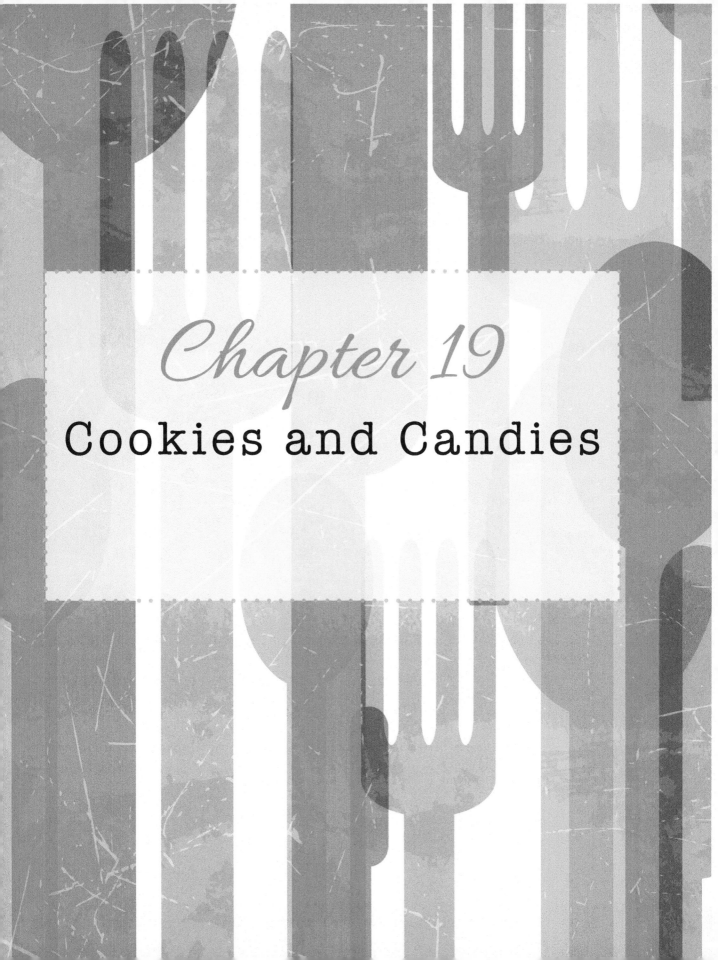

Chapter 19
Cookies and Candies

GINGERBREAD MAN COOKIES WITH GINGER AND CINNAMON OIL

Serves 20

Have fun cooking and decorating these gingerbread men made with real ginger.

RECOMMENDED ESSENTIAL OILS:

1 drop of ginger oil
1 drop of cinnamon oil

WHAT YOU WILL NEED:

1 1/2 cups flour
1 tsp. baking soda
1/4 lb. butter
3/4 cup brown sugar
1 egg
4 tbsp. golden syrup
Icing decorations
1 tsp. ground cinnamon (or 1 drop cinnamon essential oil)
2 tsp. ground ginger (or 1 drop ginger essential oil)

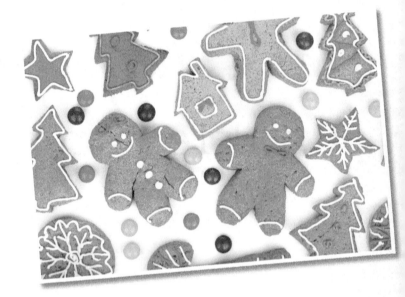

WHAT TO DO:

1. In a mixing bowl, combine the flour, baking soda, dried ginger and cinnamon.

2. Add in the butter to form crumbs.

3. Next, add in the sugar and stir well. Then, whisk the egg with the syrup and add in the ginger and cinnamon oils.

4. Add the egg mixture into the crumb mixture and transfer it into the food processor. Pulse until it all clumps together and forms into a ball.

5. Wrap dough in plastic and chill it in the fridge for about 10 to 15 minutes.

6. Preheat oven to 350 degrees and grease two cookie sheets.

7. Take the dough out from the fridge, roll it out and cut out your gingerbread men.

8. Line them up on the baking sheet and bake for 15 minutes. Let them cool completely before decorating them with the icing.

SHORTBREAD COOKIES WITH LAVENDER AND SPEARMINT OIL

Serves 24

These light shortbread cookies have a twist with lavender and mint infusions.

RECOMMENDED ESSENTIAL OILS:

1 drop of lavender oil

1 drop of spearmint oil

WHAT YOU WILL NEED:

1 1/2 cups soft butter

2/3 cup granulated sugar

1/4 cup powdered sugar

1 tsp. lemon zest

2 1/2 cups flour

1/2 cup cornstarch

1/4 tsp. salt

2 tbsp. fresh lavender (or 1 drop lavender essential oil)

1 tbsp. mint leaves (or 1 drop spearmint essential oil)

WHAT TO DO:

1. In a bowl, combine butter, granulated sugar and powdered sugar. Stir well. It will become fluffy.
2. Next, add in the flour, salt and cornstarch. Mix well.
3. Add in the lavender and mint leaves or essential oils. Combine thoroughly, then divide the dough into two balls and wrap them in plastic.
4. Flatten them out to an inch thick and refrigerate for an hour.
5. Preheat oven to 325 degrees and prepare cookie sheets. Flour a clean surface and roll the dough until it is about 1/4 of an inch thick.
6. Using a cookie cutter, cut the shapes you want. Line them up on the cookie sheet. Bake for 15-20 minutes or until the cookies become light brown. Let cookies cool before serving.

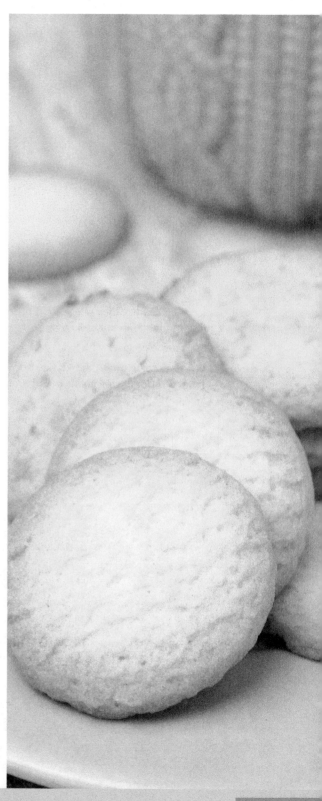

PEPPERMINT BARK WITH PEPPERMINT OIL

Serves 8-10

Perfect for the holidays, this peppermint and chocolate bark is a match made in heaven.

RECOMMENDED ESSENTIAL OILS:

1 drop of peppermint oil

WHAT YOU WILL NEED:

12 oz. dark chocolate
12 oz. white chocolate
8 peppermint candy canes
1 drop peppermint essential oil

WHAT TO DO:

1. Place the candy canes into a food processor and pulse until they are all broken up.
2. Cover a cookie sheet with foil.
3. In a saucepan, melt the dark chocolate then spread it across the foil about 1/8 of an inch thick. Place in the fridge.
4. In a another saucepan, melt the white chocolate. Add a drop of peppermint oil, along with 3/4 of the candy canes.
5. After the dark chocolate has been in the fridge for about 15 minutes, remove then spread the white chocolate mixture on the top.
6. Sprinkle the other 1/4 of the candy canes on top and make sure they are secure. Allow candy to chill in the fridge for 1 hour. Once chocolate has hardened, break into pieces. Store in an airtight bag or container.

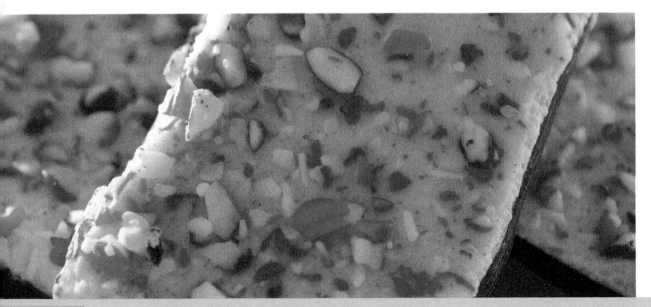

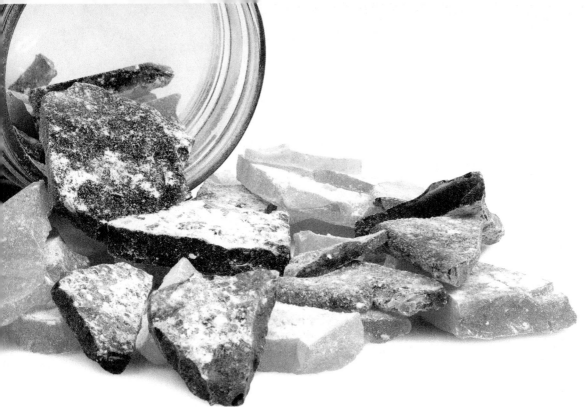

HOMEMADE HARD CANDIES WITH OIL OF YOUR CHOICE

Serves 12

Ever wonder how to make hard candies at home? Here you can - it's simple!

RECOMMENDED ESSENTIAL OILS:

Any oil flavoring of your choice (orange, lemon, lime, vanilla, peppermint, cinnamon)

WHAT YOU WILL NEED:

4 cups granulated sugar
1 cup corn syrup (light)
1 cup water
Food coloring
Confectioner's sugar

WHAT TO DO:

1. Start by covering a baking sheet with confectioner's sugar.

2. In a saucepan, combine the syrup and water, then stir until the sugar has dissolved. Once it dissolves do not touch it, but allow it to simmer for about 45 minutes.

3. Remove from the heat. For flavoring, add in your choice of 4-6 drops of essential oils. You may also want to add food coloring (optional).

4. Pour the mixture onto the cookie sheet and allow it to cool. Once cooled, place a towel on top of the hardened candy and break it with a hammer. Top with powdered sugar and enjoy. Make different batches with different essential oils and colors.

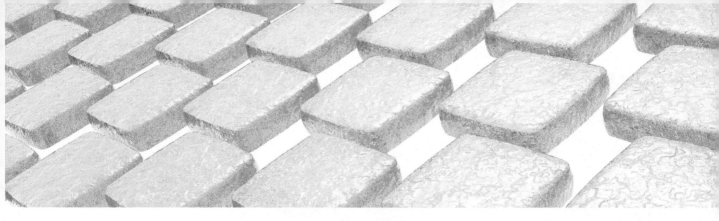

ORANGE GUMMIES WITH ORANGE OIL

Makes 40 Pieces

Who needs gummy worms when you can make these homemade orange gummies?

RECOMMENDED ESSENTIAL OILS:

1 drop of orange oil

WHAT YOU WILL NEED:

1/3 cup orange juice
1/2 cup gelatin (grass-fed)
1/4 cup raw honey
Food coloring (5 red drops, 5 yellow drops)

WHAT TO DO:

1.   Prepare a 9x9-inch pan with butter and set aside.
2.   In a saucepan, mix all of the ingredients and heat until dissolved (but do not boil).
3.   Let mixture cool to room temperature. Add in orange essential oil and any food coloring.
4.   Pour into molds and place in freezer for 15 minutes.
5.   Prepare a sheet of wax paper with sugar and invert the candy onto the wax paper. Lightly cover.
6.   Store in a cool place or refrigerate until ready to eat.

PEANUT BUTTER AND CHOCOLATE KISS COOKIES WITH VANILLA OIL

Serves 18 (36 Cookies)

This timeless classic is a delicious blend of peanut butter on the bottom and chocolate on the top, infused with vanilla oil.

RECOMMENDED ESSENTIAL OILS:

1 drop of vanilla oil

WHAT YOU WILL NEED:

1 1/2 cup flour
1/2 cup peanut butter
1/2 cup sugar
1 egg
1/2 cup butter, softened
1/2 cup brown sugar, packed
3/4 tsp. baking soda
1/2 tsp. baking powder
1 tsp. vanilla extract (and 1 drop vanilla essential oil)
24 chocolate kisses

WHAT TO DO:

1. Preheat oven to 375 degrees.
2. In a large bowl, beat sugar, brown sugar, peanut butter, butter and egg with an electric mixer on medium speed. Stir in vanilla extract and/or 1 drop of vanilla essential oil.
3. Stir in flour, baking soda and baking powder until dough forms.
4. Roll the dough into little balls and line them up on a cookie sheet. Bake for about 10 minutes (they may show slight cracks).
5. Remove from the oven and press a kiss into the middle of each cookie. Let them cool before eating.

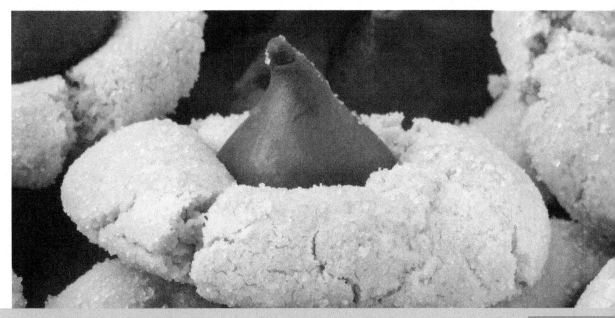

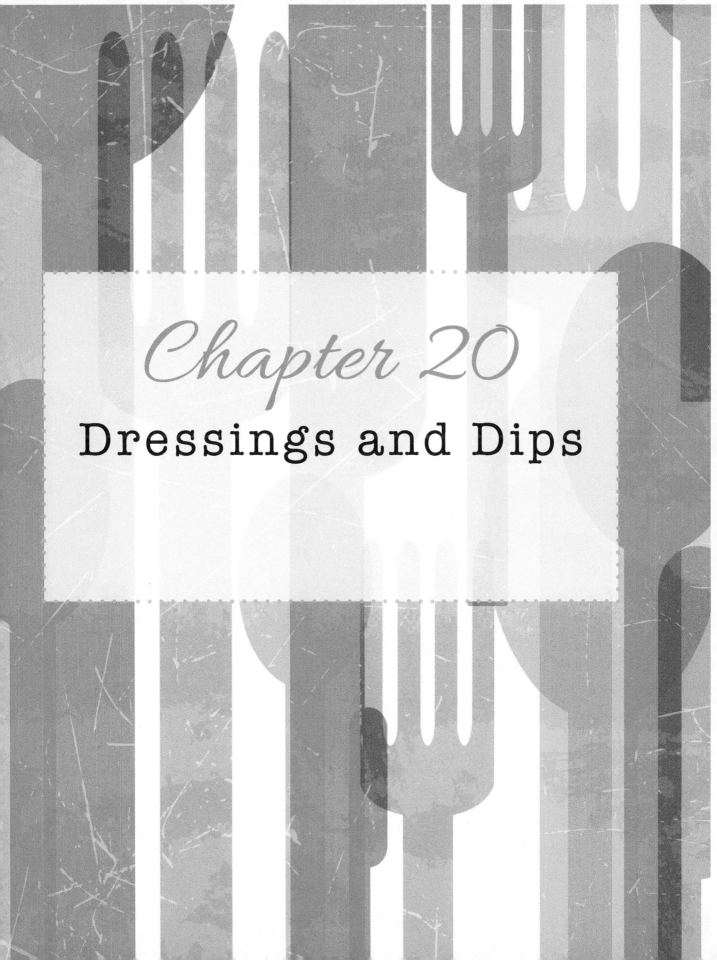

Chapter 20
Dressings and Dips

HOMEMADE RANCH DRESSING WITH PARSLEY AND DILL OIL

Make delicious creamy ranch dressing at home with real herbs.

RECOMMENDED ESSENTIAL OILS:

    3 drops of parsley oil

    1 drop of dill oil

WHAT YOU WILL NEED:

    1 clove of garlic

    1/4 tsp. salt

    1 cup mayonnaise

    1/2 cup sour cream

    1 tbsp. minced chives

    1/2 tsp. black pepper

    1/2 tsp. vinegar (white)

    1/4 tsp. paprika

    1/8 tsp. cayenne pepper

    1/4 cup buttermilk to thicken

    1/4 cup fresh parsley (or 3 drops parsley essential oil)

    2 tbsp. fresh dill, minced (or 1 drop dill essential oil)

WHAT TO DO:

1. Make a garlic paste by smashing the garlic with a fork and adding salt to it. Add this to a small bowl along with the mayonnaise, parsley oil, dill oil (or herbs if you choose), chives and sour cream.

2. Stir in the vinegar, pepper, paprika and cayenne. If you want a thicker consistency, pour in buttermilk and stir.

3. Chill in the fridge for 2 hours before serving. Adjust seasonings to your taste preference.

ITALIAN SALAD DRESSING WITH OREGANO, THYME AND BLACK PEPPER OIL

Try this classic oil and vinegar dressing filled with delicious herbs and spices.

RECOMMENDED ESSENTIAL OILS:

1 drop of parsley oil
1 drop of onion oil
1 drop of garlic oil
1 drop of oregano oil
1 drop of black pepper oil
1 drop of thyme oil
1 drop of basil oil

WHAT YOU WILL NEED:

1 cup vinegar
1 1/3 cups olive oil
2 tbsp. water
1/2 tbsp. honey
1 tbsp. sugar
1/2 tbsp. dried parsley (or 1 drop parsley essential oil)
1/2 tbsp. onion powder (or 1 drop onion essential oil)
1/2 tbsp. garlic powder (or 1 drop garlic essential oil)
1 tbsp. dried oregano (or 1 drop oregano essential oil)
1/2 tsp. ground black pepper (or 1 drop black pepper essential oil)
1/4 tsp. dried thyme (or 1 drop thyme essential oil)
1/2 tsp. dried basil (or 1 drop basil essential oil)

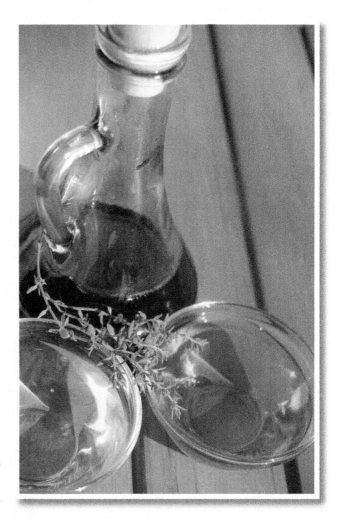

WHAT TO DO:

1. Add all ingredients (except essential oils) together in a glass jar, cover and shake well.
2. Add one or more of the essential oils, then taste test. Use the toothpick method for strong oils.
3. Will keep in the refrigerator for months.

RASPBERRY VINAIGRETTE WITH PEPPERMINT OIL

This sweet raspberry vinaigrette has a hint of mint!

RECOMMENDED ESSENTIAL OILS:

1 drop of peppermint oil

WHAT YOU WILL NEED:

1/2 cup raspberry vinegar

1 tbsp. raw honey

1 tbsp. mint leaves (or 1 drop peppermint essential oil)

WHAT TO DO:

1. Combine all ingredients in a mason jar and shake well.
2. Adjust honey to sweeten. Enjoy!

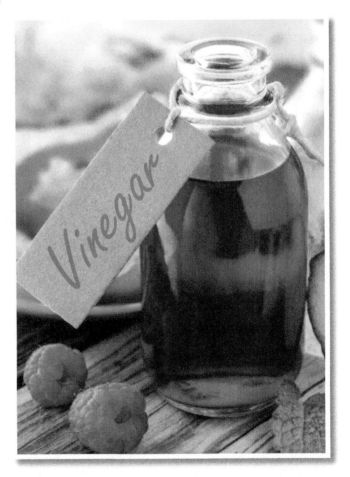

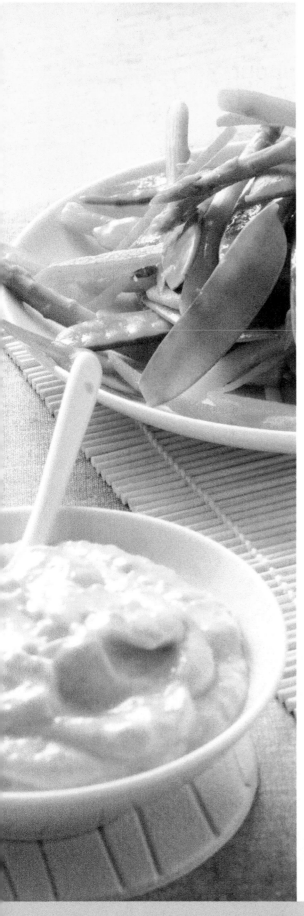

ASIAN DRESSING WITH ORANGE OIL

Switch up your salads at home with an Asian style salad dressing.

RECOMMENDED ESSENTIAL OILS:

2 drops of orange oil

WHAT YOU WILL NEED:

1/2 cup fresh orange juice (and 2 drops orange essential oil)
1/3 cup vinegar (white)
2 tbsp. sesame seeds
1 tbsp. Asian style mustard
1/4 tsp. salt
1 clove garlic, minced
3 tbsp. sesame oil

WHAT TO DO:

1. Whisk together all ingredients except the sesame oil. Stir in orange essential oil.
2. Slowly whisk the sesame oil in last. Then serve.

PESTO WITH GARLIC, BLACK PEPPER AND PARSLEY OIL

This flavorful pesto sauce is great for sandwiches!

RECOMMENDED ESSENTIAL OILS:

2 drops of parsley oil
1 drop of black pepper oil
1 drop of garlic oil

WHAT YOU WILL NEED:

1 tsp. minced garlic (and 1 drop garlic essential oil)
1/2 cup extra virgin olive oil
Salt and fresh ground black pepper to taste (or 1 drop black pepper essential oil)
1/2 cup fresh parsley, flat-leaf (and 1 drop parsley essential oil)

WHAT TO DO:

1. In a small mixing bowl, add the parsley, parsley oil, black pepper oil and garlic.
2. Gradually stir in the olive oil and add seasonings to taste. This pesto can be kept in the fridge for 3 weeks.

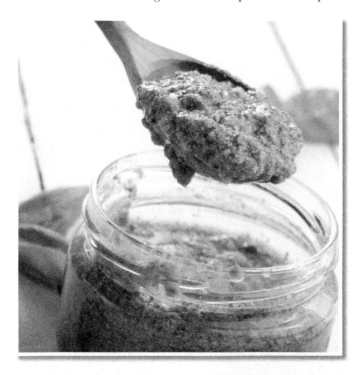

FRENCH ONION DIP WITH TARRAGON AND ROSEMARY OIL

Having a party? This creamy dip is great for dipping vegetables or potato chips.

RECOMMENDED ESSENTIAL OILS:

1 drop of rosemary oil

1 drop of tarragon oil

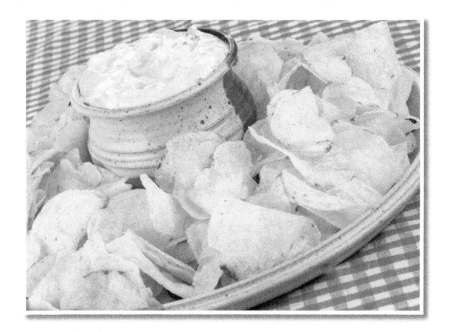

WHAT YOU WILL NEED:

1 tbsp. butter

1 tsp. olive oil

1/2 cup yellow onion, minced

Pinch of sugar

Pinch of salt

2 garlic cloves

1/4 tsp. thyme

1 tbsp. sherry vinegar

1/2 cup Greek yogurt

1 tbsp. fresh minced or
1/4 tsp. dried rosemary (or 1
drop rosemary essential oil)

1/2 tsp. dried tarragon (or 1
drop tarragon essential oil)
parsley

1 tbsp. fresh parsley, minced

WHAT TO DO:

1. In a small sauce pan, combine the butter and oil over high heat.

2. Add in the onions, salt and sugar. Allow the onions to caramelize for about 5 to 10 minutes. Next, add in the garlic and stir for 30 seconds.

3. Blend in the other herbs, spices and essential oils. Be sure to use a toothpick to dab the oil and stir it in so the flavor doesn't overpower the dip.

4. Finally, add the vinegar. Sauté until the vinegar evaporates. Then, stir the onions into the yogurt and parsley.

5. Serve or store for one week in the fridge.

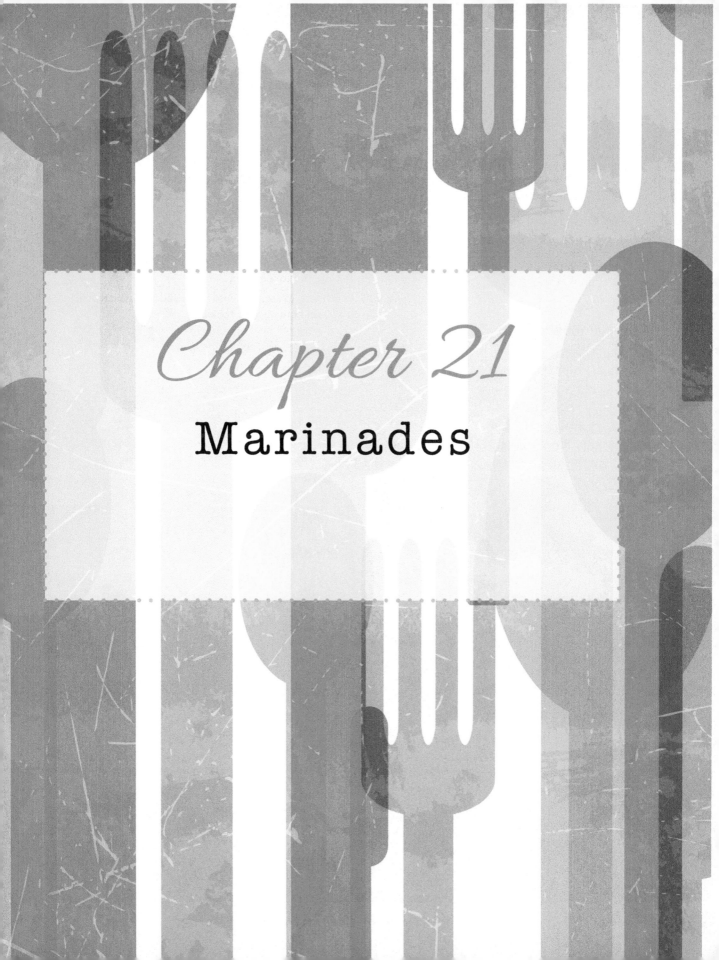

Chapter 21
Marinades

LEMON HERB MARINADE WITH LEMON AND THYME OIL

This is a great blend of lemon, basil, and thyme, which goes great on chicken or fish.

RECOMMENDED ESSENTIAL OILS:

1 drop of basil oil
1 drop of thyme oil

WHAT YOU WILL NEED:

1 cup olive oil
1/4 cup lemon juice
1/4 tsp. salt
1/4 tsp. pepper
2 garlic cloves, chopped
1 tbsp. fresh basil (and 1 drop basil essential oil)
1/2 tsp. dried thyme (and 1 drop thyme essential oil)

WHAT TO DO:

1. Mix all of the ingredients together and store in a glass jar in the fridge up to a month.
2. When ready to use, pour into a dish and add meat to marinade for several hours before cooking.

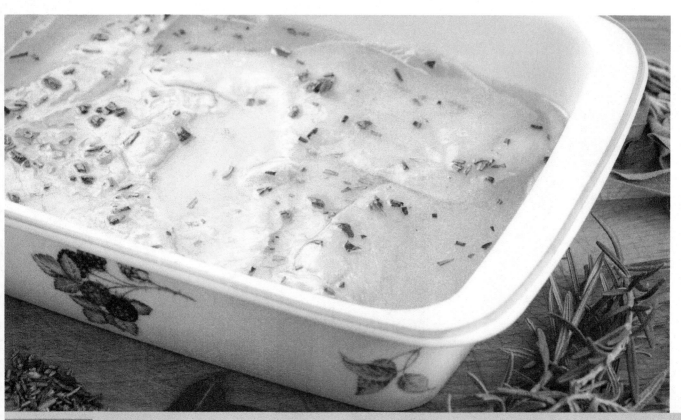

HERB MARINADE WITH GARLIC AND SAVORY OIL

Garlic herb marinade is great for any kind of entrée. Very versatile!

RECOMMENDED ESSENTIAL OILS:

2 drops of savory oil
1 drop of garlic oil

WHAT YOU WILL NEED:

2 tbsp. rice vinegar
1 tsp. extra virgin olive oil
1 lemon for zest, wedges for garnish
Salt and pepper to taste
4 tbsp. dried savory (or 2 drops savory essential oil)
1 tsp. garlic, coarsely chopped (or 1 drop garlic essential oil)

WHAT TO DO:

1. In a container, combine all of the ingredients together. Shake well to blend.
2. Brush onto meat and let sit for several hours before cooking.

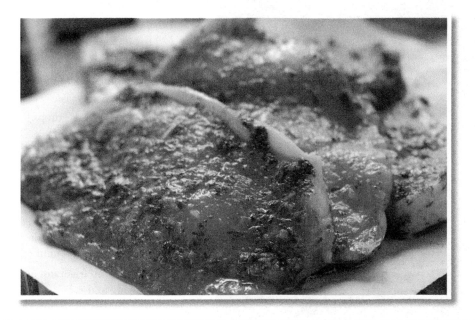

Tip:
Try brushing on marjoram-flavored olive oil when barbecuing meat or kebabs on the grill.

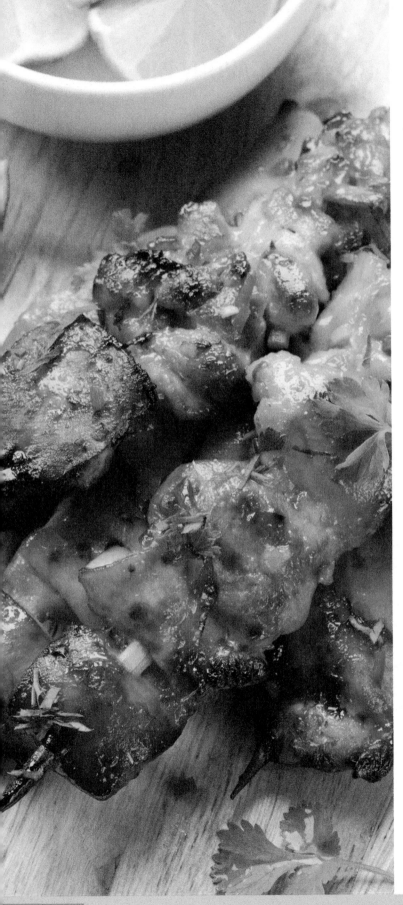

CILANTRO MARINADE WITH LIME AND CUMIN OIL

A delicious combination of cilantro and lime, ideal for grilling chicken.

RECOMMENDED ESSENTIAL OILS:

2 drops of lime oil

1 drop of cumin oil

WHAT YOU WILL NEED:

1/3 cup olive oil

1 garlic clove

1 tbsp. fresh cilantro

1/2 tsp. chili powder

2 tsp. sugar

1/2 tsp. red pepper flakes

Salt and pepper to taste

2 limes, juiced (and 2 drops lime essential oil)

1/2 tsp. ground cumin (or 1 drop cumin essential oil)

WHAT TO DO:

1. Combine all the ingredients in a food processor and blend until well combined.

2. Store in the refrigerator in a glass bottle until ready to use.

JAMAICAN JERK MARINADE WITH NUTMEG AND THYME OIL

Get a little taste of paradise to make you feel like you're somewhere tropical with this Jamaican jerk marinade.

RECOMMENDED ESSENTIAL OILS:

1 drop of thyme oil
1 drop of nutmeg oil

WHAT YOU WILL NEED:

1 medium onion, finely chopped
1/2 cup scallions, finely chopped
1 hot pepper, finely chopped
3 tbsp. soy sauce
1 tbsp. oil
1 tbsp. cider vinegar
2 tsp. sugar

1 tsp. salt
1 tsp. ground Jamaican Pimento (allspice)
1 tsp. black pepper
1/2 tsp. ground cinnamon
2 tsp. fresh thyme (and 1 drop thyme essential oil)
1/2 tsp. ground nutmeg (or 1 drop nutmeg essential oil)

WHAT TO DO:

1. Combine all ingredients together in a food processor. Pulse to blend together.
2. Store in the refrigerator for up to 2 months. Use to marinade meat before grilling.

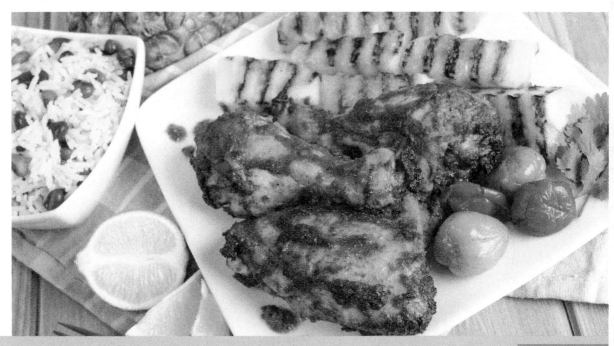

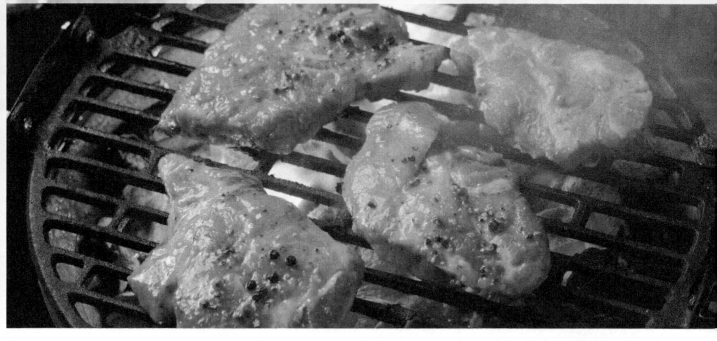

STEAK MARINADE WITH OREGANO AND BLACK PEPPER OIL

Makes about 3/4 cup

A classic marinade that is great for steaks.

RECOMMENDED ESSENTIAL OILS:

1 drop of oregano oil
1 drop of black pepper oil

WHAT YOU WILL NEED:

1/4 cup cooking oil
1/4 cup red wine vinegar
3 tbsp. Worcestershire sauce
1 tbsp. salt
1 tsp. dried thyme
1 tsp. dried oregano (or 1 drop oregano essential oil)
1 tsp. ground black pepper (or 1 drop black pepper essential oil)

WHAT TO DO:

1. In a glass jar or container, combine all of the ingredients. Mix well.
2. Store in the refrigerator until ready for use (up to a month).

PINEAPPLE MARINADE WITH GINGER OIL

RECOMMENDED ESSENTIAL OILS:

    1 drop of ginger oil

WHAT YOU WILL NEED:

    1 cup crushed pineapple
    1/3 cup soy sauce
    1/3 cup honey
    1/4 cup cider vinegar
    2 cloves garlic, minced
    1 tsp. ginger powder (or 1 drop ginger essential oil)
    1/4 tsp. powdered cloves

WHAT TO DO:

1. Mix all ingredients together and refrigerate.
2. Store in an airtight container for up to 7 days.

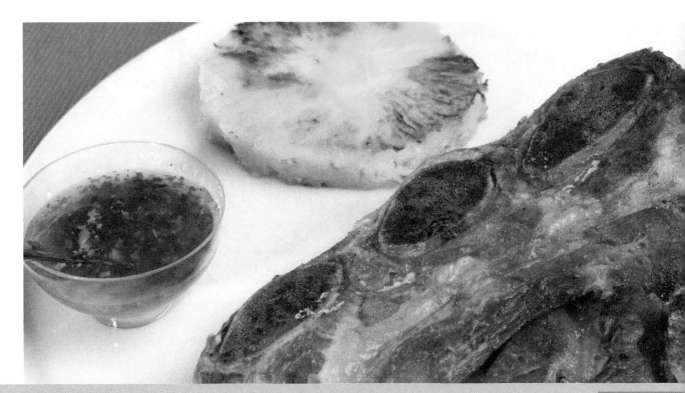

DIPPING OIL

Makes 2 cups

Make your own herbed infused dipping oil customized to your tastes with your favorite herbs!

RECOMMENDED ESSENTIAL OILS:

Add your favorite essential oil

WHAT YOU WILL NEED:

2 cups olive oil
2 tbsp. Parmesan cheese
1 tbsp. dried basil
1 tbsp. dried parsley
1 tbsp. garlic, minced
1 tsp. dried thyme
1 tsp. dried oregano
1 tsp. ground black pepper
1/2 tsp. dried rosemary, crushed
1/2 tsp. salt
1/2 tsp. red pepper, crushed
1/2 tsp. lemon juice

WHAT TO DO:

1. Combine all the herbs and oil together.
2. Add in the lemon juice, essential oils of choice and stir. Taste and adjust accordingly.
3. Sprinkle parmesan cheese on the top.

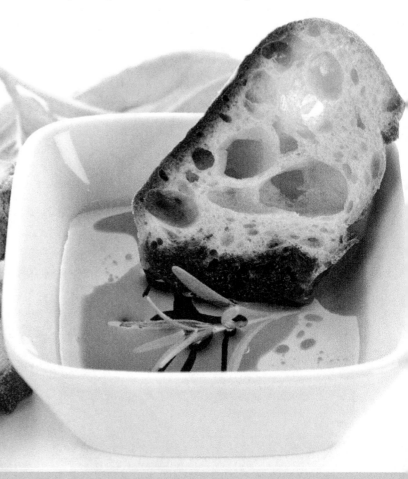

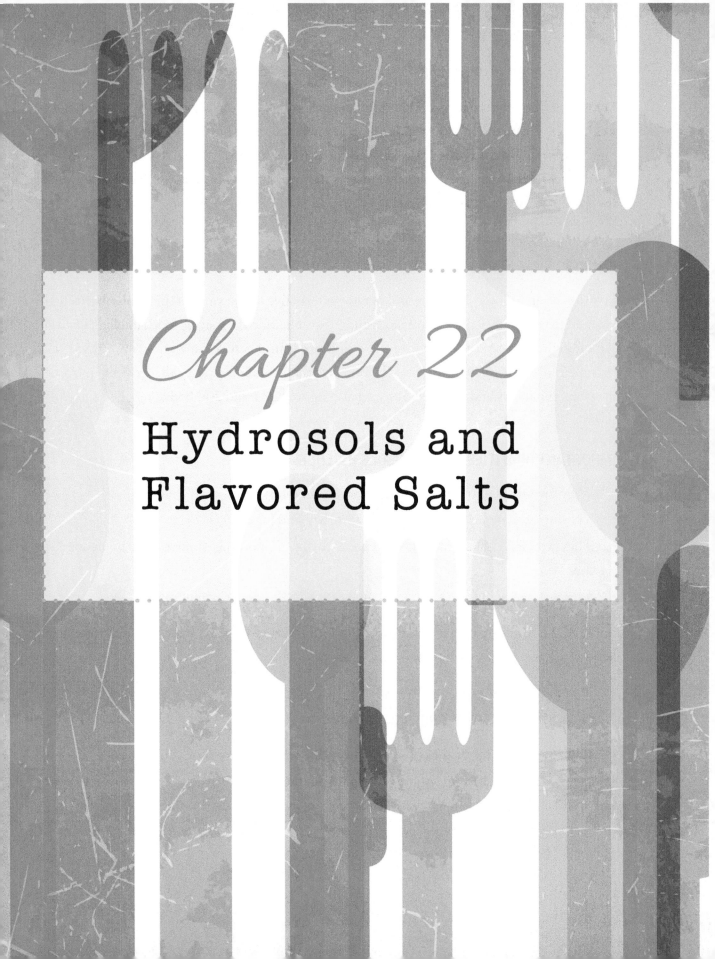

Chapter 22

Hydrosols and Flavored Salts

USING HYDROSOLS IN COOKING

Hydrosols, also referred to as herbal distillates, are colloidal suspensions or aqueous solutions made from essential oils by steam distilling aromatic plants. They are known by many other names such as herbal water, hydrolate, essential water or floral water. These hydrosols are commonly used in skin care, medicine and as flavorings. Some examples include rose water, orange flower water and witch hazel.

COOKING WITH HYDROSOLS

Hydrosols can become a vibrant and healthy alternative to the various spices and herbs that you add to your daily food. Essential oils and hydrosols added to specific foods intelligently will not only stimulate your taste buds but also improve your digestive capabilities. Your food will become more flavorful and fragrant. Hydrosols, when combined to meals, serve the purpose of flavor enhancers and aphrodisiacs, and also rejuvenate mind and body.

IMPORTANT QUALITIES OF HYDROSOLS INCLUDE:

- They are 30-40% stronger in comparison to an infusion
- They are water-soluble; hence, easily absorbed and ingested
- They are very much diluted, sometimes to the proportions similar to a homeopathic medicine
- They are very gentle on the body, but are highly effective or potent in their action

Some of the plants that make great hydrosols include lavender, sage, rose, oregano, rosemary, lemon verbena, rose geranium, mint and hyssop.

WAYS YOU CAN USE HYDROSOLS IN COOKING:

- Replace all or some of the water in your recipe with a hydrosol of your choice
- Freeze the hydrosols into ice cube trays and put these flavored hydrosol ice cubes into your drinks and water for an excellent flavor.

Some examples of hydrosols that you can use in your everyday cooking include:

Lemon Balm hydrosol: This hydrosol can be added while preparing food punches or on lamb. You can make a refreshing drink by adding lemon verbena hydrosols to water.

Rosemary hydrosol: This hydrosol can either be added to a marinade or sprinkled on poultry that imparts an excellent savory flavor.

Peppermint hydrosol: You can freeze peppermint hydrosols in ice cube trays and place the ice cubes into iced tea making a cooling and refreshing summer drink. You can also add these ice cubes to glasses of lemonade to impart excellent flavor to the drink.

Lavender hydrosol: This hydrosol can also be added to teas to make a great tasting drink. Lavender hydrosol can also be used to prepare vinegars for salads or marinades. You can add lavender hydrosols to your cookie recipe to impart a floral and lemony flavor to them.

Oregano hydrosol: You can freeze oregano hydrosol in ice cube trays and use these in tomato juice to divulge an excellent flavor.

Hydrosols are an excellent alternative to using essential oils in your cooking. Being water soluble, they are easily ingested and absorbed. Increase the flavor of your recipes by adding your choice of hydrosols into your daily meals and get the benefit of health, too!

FLAVORED SALTS

Salt adds a little something to a dish that makes it just right. You can take that addition to the next level by infusing salts with different flavors and essential oils. Many people are familiar with seasoned salt or garlic salt that can be purchased at the grocery store. But, did you know you can make your own salts with a much larger variety right at home using dried herbs, fruits, essential oils and more? When made at home they don't contain any of the harmful chemicals or anti-caking agents that store-bought seasonings contain in order to keep their shelf life. In fact, salt crystals can extract and absorb essential oils and flavors from herbs with no effort and no special equipment. Famous chefs such as Sara Jenkins, owner of Porchetta, sells *Porchetta Salt*, created with tasty Mediterranean herbs and wild fennel pollen. Dario Cecchini, a butcher and restaurant owner in Tuscany, Italy, has packed aroma from lavender, bay leaves, thyme and rosemary into an ultrafine Italian sea salt called, *Profumo del Chianti*.

There are many possibilities to the flavors of salt you can make, along with multiple ways you can use them. When these flavored salts are made fresh with natural ingredients, the quality of flavor is in a league of its own. They can be used as table seasoning, on the grill or in other cooking. Listed below are some of the ways to use seasoned salts, with flavor ideas for making them and a list of recipes to get you started.

HOW SALTS CAN BE USED

The possibilities for flavors are far reaching. Get creative! Here are a few ideas of how to use seasoned salts in your cooking.

The rim of cocktail glasses (great for martinis)	Corn on the cob
French fries	Salad dressings
Grilled meats	Guacamole
Scrambled eggs	Fried foods
Popcorn	Seafood
Bruschetta	Hamburgers
Roasted vegetables	Ribs
Sliced tomatoes	Chops
Soups	Grilled fish or chicken
Stew	

FLAVOR IDEAS

Here are some flavor families to get you started, but don't be afraid to experiment and create your own blend.

SWEET OR FLORAL HERBS

Lavender
Lemon balm
Lemon verbena
Rose
Dill
Mint
Nutmeg

SAVORY HERBS

Marjoram
Oregano
Parsley
Savory
Tarragon
Thyme
Bay leaf

ROBUST HERBS

- Rosemary
- Sage
- Basil
- Cilantro

SPICES

- Cinnamon
- Pepper

DEHYDRATED FRUITS OR VEGETABLES

- Celery
- Mushrooms
- Garlic
- Ginger
- Lemon
- Lime
- Onion
- Orange
- Chile Peppers

CITRUS ZEST

- Grapefruit
- Lemon
- Lime
- Orange

HERB SEEDS

- Whole caraway
- Celery
- Coriander
- Cumin
- Fennel
- Poppy
- Sesame

FOR PREPARING YOUR SEASONED SALTS

The base of each combination is salt. It is recommended to use additive-free salt or fine sea salt depending on the recipe. Good brands to look for are kosher, Maldon or fleur de sel. Once you have your salt, there are a few other items you will want to pick up. You will want a small, medium or large jar depending on the quantity you want to keep on hand. It is best to have both breathable containers and airtight containers. Humid conditions may vary according to the climate where you live, therefore where moisture is found, you may want a breathable container so that moisture doesn't get trapped. Follow the below for drying out the salts.

The following tools will come in handy: toothpicks, measuring spoons and cups, an oven, a food processor and baking sheet.

The flavorings that you choose should be dried and chopped into very small pieces. For any wet ingredients (such as citrus peels or fresh herbs) dry those in an oven that is set on low heat (about 150-200 degrees). You can also use a dehydrator.

When using the essential oils you have on hand, you can use the toothpick method to mix the oils in. Start by dipping the toothpick into a drop of the oil and then stir it into the salt mixture. Taste test as you mix to get the flavor just right.

Once you have all of your tools ready, here is a general method to make the salts:

1. Take 1/4 cup of salt and add it to the container.

2. Next, choose the dried or oil flavoring that you want and start by mixing in 1 teaspoon or use the toothpick method for essential oil. You can gradually add in more flavoring, taste testing it as you go along.

3. Use your food processor to pulse the ingredients together, but be careful not to fully pulverize the salt.

4. If the mix is completely moisture free, store it in an airtight container. It can keep for up to a year.

5. If you find the salt is moist, store it in a breathable container or spread it out on a dish and place it in direct sunlight. Or, store the salt in a loosely sealed bag and place it in the

freezer for 12 hours to freeze-dry the outside edges of the salt crystals. Another option is to spread the mixed salt onto a baking sheet and heat the oven to warm (under 250 degrees to preserve the minerals in the salt). Once warm, turn off the oven and place baking sheet in oven. Allow it to sit until you are satisfied with the dryness.

LEMON PEPPER SEASONING

Makes 1/2 cup

This seasoning brings vibrant flavors unlike any lemon pepper seasoning you have picked up from the store. It goes great with fish, seafood and poultry.

RECOMMENDED ESSENTIAL OILS:

1 drop of lemon oil
1 drop of black pepper oil

WHAT YOU WILL NEED:

4 tbsp. dried lemon peel (or 1 drop lemon essential oil)
2 tbsp. black peppercorns (and 1 drop black pepper essential oil)
3 tsp. finely ground sea salt
1 tsp. citric acid

WHAT TO DO:

1. Process the lemon peel and pepper in a food processor until fine, then stir in the black pepper oil and lemon oil.
2. Once mixed well, add in the salt and citric acid.
3. Combine all the ingredients together and use the drying process if needed.
4. Place into a storage container.

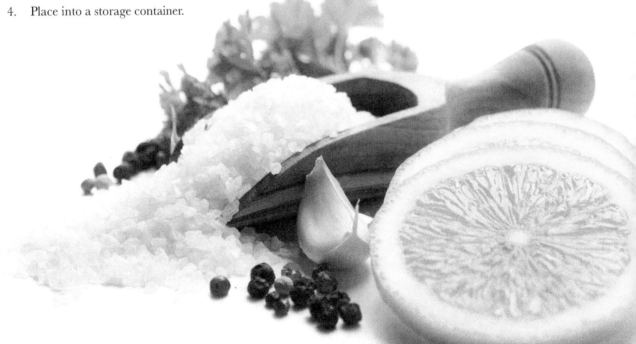

CLASSIC SEASONING SALT

Makes 1/3 cup

This seasoning salt is packed with flavors and is even cheaper to make than to buy premade. Add this seasoning salt to hamburgers, meat, popcorn or corn on the cob.

RECOMMENDED ESSENTIAL OILS:

- 1 drop of onion oil
- 1 drop of garlic oil
- 1 drop of celery seed oil

WHAT YOU WILL NEED:

- 4 tbsp. finely ground sea salt
- 2 tsp. paprika
- 1/2 tsp. turmeric
- 1/2 tsp. onion powder (or 1 drop onion essential oil)
- 1/2 tsp. garlic powder (or 1 drop garlic essential oil)
- 1/2 tsp. celery seed (or 1 drop celery seed essential oil)
- 1/2 tsp. ground cumin

WHAT TO DO:

1. Finely grind all your ingredients using a food processor, stir in the essential oils using the toothpick method and dry herbs, if needed.

2. Pour the salt blend into a container for storage.

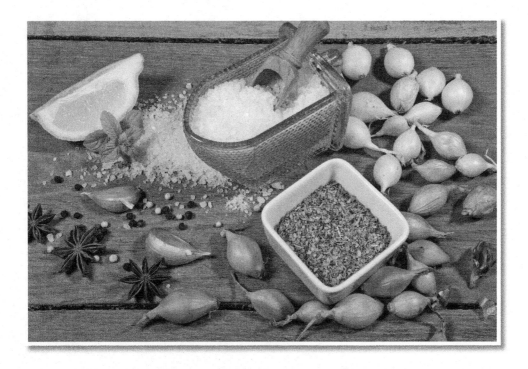

TACO SEASONING

Makes 3/4 cup

Here is a homemade replacement for that envelope of taco seasoning. This mix can be used in a variety of Mexican style dishes including taco meat, rice, burrito meat and other dinner dishes.

RECOMMENDED ESSENTIAL OILS:

1 drop of garlic oil
1 drop of onion oil
1 drop of oregano oil
1 drop of cumin oil

WHAT TO DO:

1. Dry and process all of the ingredients in a food processor.
2. Mix in essential oils using the toothpick method, if desired.
3. Store in a container until ready for use. It will keep for 2 to 3 months.

WHAT YOU WILL NEED:

1/4 cup chili powder
1 tsp. garlic powder (or 1 drop garlic essential oil)
1 tsp. onion powder (or 1 drop onion essential oil)
1 tsp. crushed red pepper flakes
1 tsp. dried oregano (or 1 drop oregano essential oil)
2 tsp. paprika
2 tbsp. ground cumin (or 1 drop cumin essential oil)
1 tbsp. coarse sea salt
2 tsp. black pepper
2 tbsp. arrowroot powder

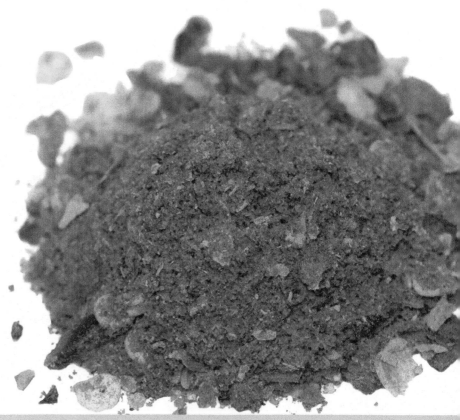

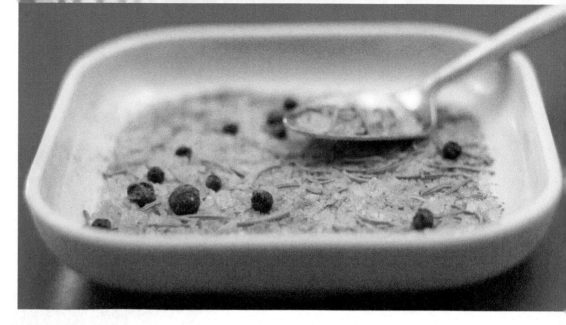

OLD BAY SEASONING

Makes 1/4 cup

This is just like the Old Bay seasoning you know and love but better. This seasoning goes great with fish, especially salmon and crab. Try this out in your crab and salmon cakes. Also try this on chicken before heating it on the grill.

RECOMMENDED ESSENTIAL OILS:

- 1 drop of celery seed oil
- 1 drop of bay leaf oil
- 1 drop of black pepper oil
- 1 drop of nutmeg oil
- 1 drop of cinnamon oil
- 1 drop of clove oil

WHAT YOU WILL NEED:

- 2 tsp. celery seeds (and 1 drop celery seed essential oil)
- 8 bay leaves (or 1 drop bay leaf essential oil)
- 2 tsp. black peppercorns (or 1 drop black pepper essential oil)
- 2 tsp. unrefined sea salt
- 2 tsp. paprika
- 1 tsp. dry mustard
- 1/8 tsp. ground nutmeg (or 1 drop nutmeg essential oil)
- 1/8 tsp. ground cinnamon (and 1 drop cinnamon essential oil)
- 1/8 tsp. ground cloves (and 1 drop clove essential oil)

WHAT TO DO:

1. In a food processor, add celery seeds, bay leaves, and peppercorns. Grind up.
2. Add the remaining ingredients and stir in any essential oils using the toothpick method.
3. On a cookie sheet, spread out salt mixture to dry, if needed.
4. Store in a container until ready to use. Will keep for 2 to 3 months.

CHILI POWDER

Makes 1/3 cup

Give your homemade chili a burst of flavor with this chili powder. It also goes great on chicken and meat dishes as well as in soups and stews.

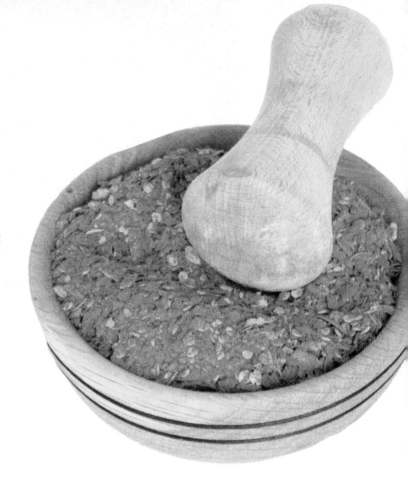

RECOMMENDED ESSENTIAL OILS:

1 drop of cumin oil
1 drop of garlic oil

WHAT YOU WILL NEED:

3 tbsp. paprika
1 tbsp. ground cumin (or 1 drop cumin essential oil)
2 tsp. dried Mexican oregano
1 tsp. cayenne pepper ground
1/2 tsp. garlic powder (and 1 drop garlic essential oil)

WHAT TO DO:

1. In a container, mix all of the ingredients well. Stir in any essential oils, using the toothpick method. Allow to dry.
2. Place in an airtight container, and store in a cool, dark place. Will last for several months.

LEMON OR LIME SALTS

Makes 1/2 cup

Dip the rim of a cocktail glass in water then lime salt for a margarita or lemon salt for an ice-cold beer. These salts can also be used with desserts.

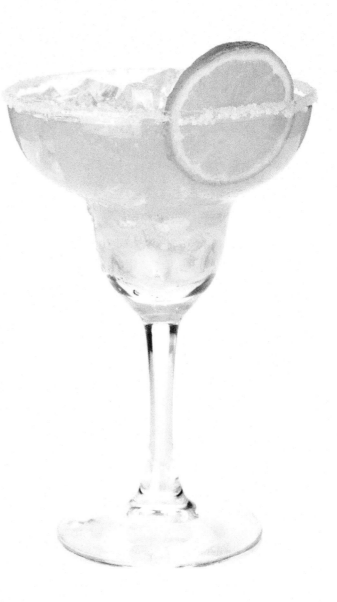

RECOMMENDED ESSENTIAL OILS:

1 drop of lemon oil
1 drop of lime oil

WHAT YOU WILL NEED:

1/2 cup sea salt
1 tbsp. lemon and/or lime zest (and 1-2 drops lemon or lime essential oil)

WHAT TO DO:

1. Grate the zest from the citrus fruit you choose and add essential oils in. Allow to dry.
2. Mix in with the salt thoroughly and store in an airtight container.

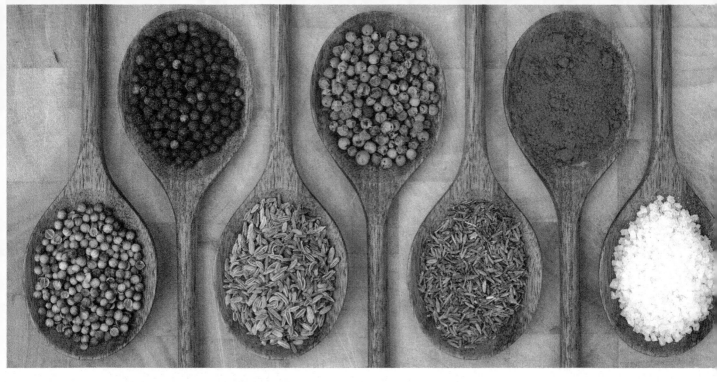

CAJUN SEASONING

Makes about 1 1/2 cups

This seasoning will add some heat to casserole dishes, eggs, chicken, and stir frys.

RECOMMENDED ESSENTIAL OILS:

1 drop of black pepper oil
1 drop of onion oil
1 drop of oregano oil
1 drop of thyme oil

WHAT YOU WILL NEED:

1/2 cup paprika
13/ cup sea salt
1/4 cup garlic powder
2 tbsp. ground black pepper (or 1 drop black pepper essential oil)
2 tbsp. onion powder (or 1 drop onion essential oil)
1 tbsp. cayenne pepper
2 tbsp. dried oregano (or 1 drop oregano essential oil)
1 tbsp. dried thyme (or 1 drop thyme essential oil)

WHAT TO DO:

1. In a processor, grind garlic, onion, sea salt and thyme together.
2. Mix in any essential oils using the toothpick method. Let dry.
3. Store blend in an airtight container.

FAJITA SEASONING

Makes about 1/2 cup

When warming up tortillas and stirring the guacamole, this seasoning adds great flavor and dimension to chicken, steak or shrimp in fajitas.

RECOMMENDED ESSENTIAL OILS:

1 drop of onion oil
1 drop of garlic oil

WHAT YOU WILL NEED:

1/4 cup chili powder
2 tbsp. sea salt
2 tbsp. paprika
1 tbsp. onion powder or chives (or 1 drop onion essential oil)
1 tbsp. garlic powder or minced garlic (or 1 drop garlic essential oil)
1 tsp. cayenne powder
1 tbsp. cumin ground

WHAT TO DO:

1. In a bowl, add all dry ingredients and mix well.
2. Add essential oil if desired, stirring in using the toothpick method.
3. All the mixture to dry. Store in a container until ready to use.

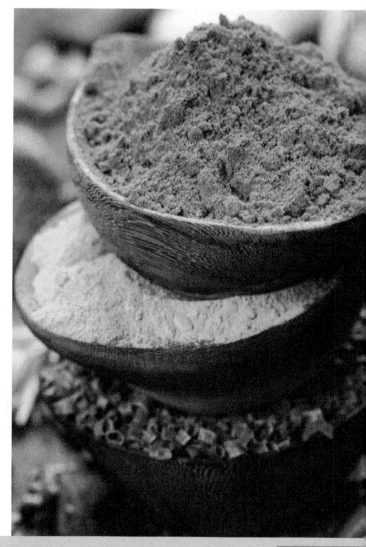

ASIAN SPICE

Makes 1/2 cup

Try this spice sautéed with beef and broccoli, on chow mein noodles or mixed into rice.

RECOMMENDED ESSENTIAL OILS:

    1 drop of black pepper oil
    1 drop of cinnamon oil
    1 drop of clove oil
    1 drop of fennel oil

WHAT YOU WILL NEED:

    2 tbsp. anise powder
    1 tbsp. black pepper (or 1 drop black pepper essential oil)
    1 tbsp. ground fennel (or 1 drop fennel essential oil)
    1 tbsp. ground cinnamon (or 1 drop cinnamon essential oil)
    1 tbsp. ground cloves (or 1 drop clove essential oil)
    1 tbsp. sea salt

WHAT TO DO:

1.   Combine all dried ingredients in the food processor and mix well.
2.   Add salt and essential oils and dry if needed. Store in a container.

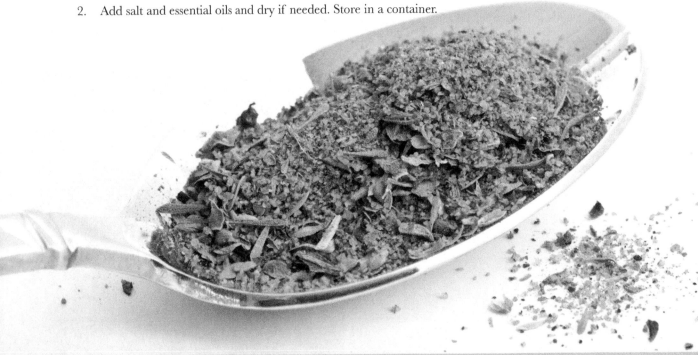

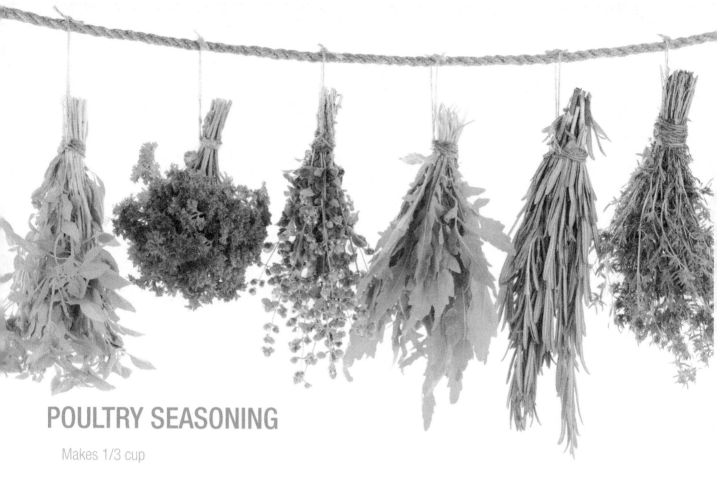

POULTRY SEASONING

Makes 1/3 cup

This seasoning is wonderful on chicken slow cooked in the crockpot. It also goes great on fall vegetables and stuffing.

RECOMMENDED ESSENTIAL OILS:

- 1 drop of rosemary oil
- 1 drop of oregano oil
- 1 drop of ginger oil
- 1 drop of marjoram oil
- 1 drop of thyme oil
- 1 drop of sage oil

WHAT YOU WILL NEED:

- 1 tbsp. dried rosemary (or 1 drop rosemary essential oil)
- 1 tbsp. dried oregano (or 1 drop oregano essential oil)
- 1 tbsp. ginger (or 1 drop ginger essential oil)
- 1 tbsp. dried marjoram (or 1 drop marjoram essential oil)
- 1 tbsp. dried thyme (or 1 drop thyme essential oil)
- 1 tsp. ground black pepper
- 1 tsp. sea salt
- 2 tbsp. dried sage (or 1 drop sage essential oil)

WHAT TO DO:

1. In a bowl or food processor, add all dry ingredients and blend together.
2. Add any essential oils using the toothpick method. Stir well to mix.
3. Let dry and store in a container until ready to use.

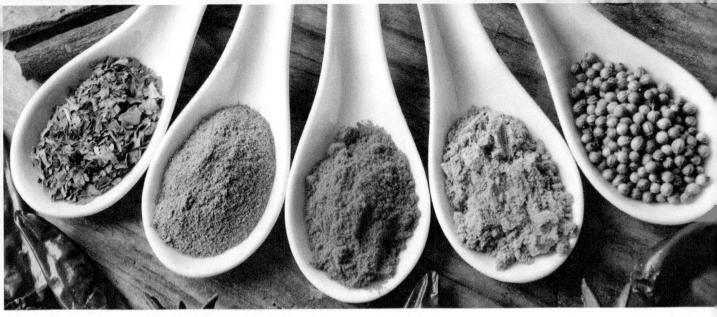

BLACKENED SPICE

Makes 1 1/2 ounces

This spice goes wonderfully on white fish or chicken. Adjust the cayenne pepper to your heat preference or for sensitive taste buds.

RECOMMENDED ESSENTIAL OILS:

1 drop of basil oil
1 drop of thyme oil
1 drop of garlic oil
1 drop of black pepper oil
1 drop of onion oil

WHAT TO DO:

1. In a bowl or food processor, add dry ingredients (except salt) and blend.
2. Add any essential oils, using the toothpick method. Let dry.
3. Add sea salt and place in a container ready for use.

WHAT YOU WILL NEED:

1 tsp. dried basil (or 1 drop basil essential oil)
1 tsp. dried thyme (or 1 drop thyme essential oil)
1 tsp. garlic powder (or 1 drop garlic essential oil)
1 tsp. white pepper
1 tsp. black pepper (or 1 drop black pepper essential oil)
1 tsp. sea salt
1 tsp. onion powder (or 1 drop onion essential oil)
2 tsp. cayenne pepper
1 tsp. paprika

ALL PURPOSE SPICE

Makes 1 1/2 ounces

This spice is great for a variety of uses; try it on meat, poultry and fish.

RECOMMENDED ESSENTIAL OILS:

1 drop of cumin oil
1 drop of coriander oil
1 drop of ginger oil

WHAT YOU WILL NEED:

4 tsp. chili powder
1/2 tsp. cumin (or 1 drop cumin essential oil)
1/2 tsp. ground coriander (or 1 drop coriander essential oil)
1/2 tsp. ground ginger (or 1 drop ginger essential oil)
1/4 tsp. Chinese five spice powder
2 tsp. coarse salt

WHAT TO DO:

1. In a bowl or processor, add all of the dry ingredients, except the salt. Blend well.
2. Add the essential oils using the toothpick method that you choose and dry the mixture if needed.
3. Mix in the salt and store in a container for future uses.

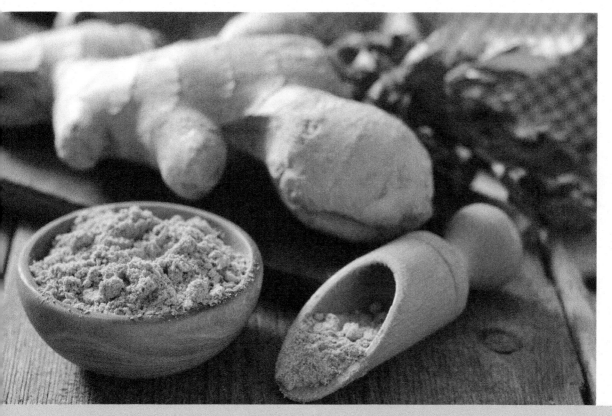

HERB SEASONING

Makes 2 ounces

This delicious spice is great on vegetables, meat, fish, and even in olive oil for dipping.

RECOMMENDED ESSENTIAL OILS:

1 drop of garlic oil

1 drop of basil oil

1 drop of marjoram oil

1 drop of thyme oil

1 drop of parsley oil

1 drop of savory oil

1 drop of onion oil

1 drop of black pepper oil

1 drop of sage oil

WHAT YOU WILL NEED:

1 tbsp. garlic powder (or 1 drop garlic essential oil)

1/2 tsp. cayenne pepper

1 tsp. dried basil (or 1 drop basil essential oil)

1 tsp. dried marjoram (or 1 drop marjoram essential oil)

1 tsp. dried thyme (or 1 drop thyme essential oil)

1 tsp. dried parsley (or 1 drop parsley essential oil)

1 tsp. dried savory (or 1 drop savory essential oil)

1 tsp. ground mace

1 tsp. onion powder (or 1 drop onion essential oil)

1 tsp. black pepper (or 1 drop black pepper essential oil)

1 tsp. ground sage (or 1 drop sage essential oil)

1 tsp. salt

WHAT TO DO:

1. Prepare all your herbs by drying them and processing them into small pieces.

2. Stir in any essential oils that you are going to include using the toothpick method.

3. Dry the mixture if needed. Combine with salt and store in a container.

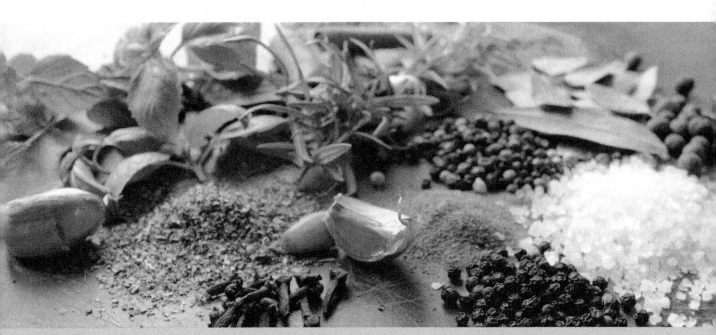

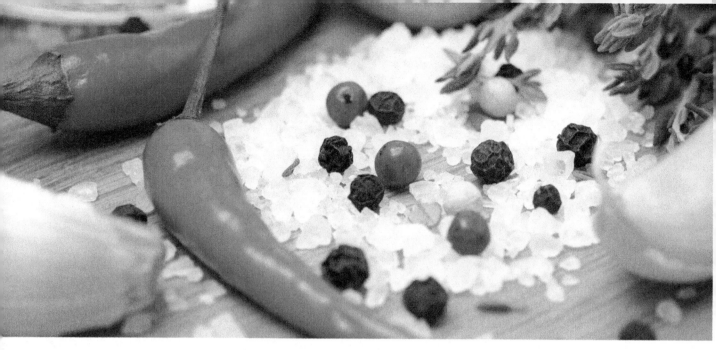

ITALIAN SPICES

Makes 3/4 cup

Use this spice to add an Italian flair to pasta sauce, sausage dishes and vinaigrette. You can also sprinkle over chicken before baking or grilling it.

RECOMMENDED ESSENTIAL OILS:

1 drop of basil oil
1 drop of marjoram oil
1 drop of garlic oil
1 drop of thyme oil
1 drop of rosemary oil
1 drop of oregano oil

WHAT YOU WILL NEED:

2 tbsp. dried basil (or 1 drop basil essential oil)
2 tbsp. dried marjoram (or 1 drop marjoram essential oil)
1 tbsp. garlic powder (or 1 drop garlic essential oil)
1 tbsp. dried oregano (or 1 drop oregano essential oil)
1 tbsp. dried thyme (or 1 drop thyme essential oil)
1 tbsp. dried rosemary (or 1 drop rosemary essential oil)
1 tbsp. crushed red pepper flakes
1 tbsp. sea salt

WHAT TO DO:

1. Prepare all the herbs by drying them (if using fresh) and add to a processor to grind and blend together.
2. Stir in the essential oils using the toothpick method.
3. Combine salt with herbs and store in an airtight container until ready to use.

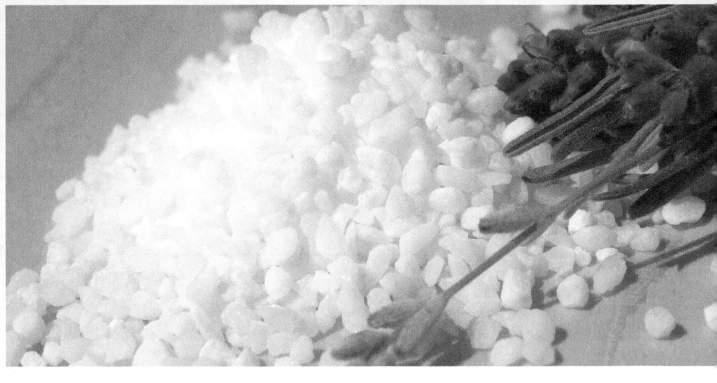

LAVENDER SALT

Makes 1/2 cup

This salt can add a nice touch to chocolate desserts. You can also try sprinkling it on freshly baked bread, potatoes or winter squash.

RECOMMENDED ESSENTIAL OILS:

1 drop of lavender oil

WHAT YOU WILL NEED:

1/2 tsp. fresh English lavender buds (and 1 drop lavender essential oil)
1/2 cup fine grey sea salt

WHAT TO DO:

1. Remove lavender buds from the stems and measure 1/2 teaspoon out to mix into the salt. Dried lavender may be substituted if fresh is unavailable.
2. Add the lavender essential oil using the toothpick method into the mixture. Allow to dry.
3. Store salt in an airtight jar until ready to use.

HEALTHY COOKING WITH ESSENTIAL OIL

TUSCAN SEASONING BLEND

Makes about 1 cup

This seasoning is inspired by the flavors in Tuscany and goes great sprinkled on chicken thighs, salmon steaks and lamb chops.

RECOMMENDED ESSENTIAL OILS:

1 drop of basil oil
1 drop of garlic oil
1 drop of rosemary oil
1 drop of oregano oil

WHAT TO DO:

1. Coarsely grind the fennel seeds and combine them with the other seasonings.
2. Stir in the oils that you would like to use and allow the mixture to dry if needed.
3. Store in an airtight container.

WHAT YOU WILL NEED:

1 tbsp. fennel seeds
6 tbsp. dried basil (and 1 drop basil essential oil)
3 tbsp. garlic powder (and 1 drop garlic essential oil)
3 tbsp. coarse salt
2 tbsp. dried rosemary (and 1 drop rosemary essential oil)
2 tbsp. dried oregano (and 1 drop oregano essential oil)

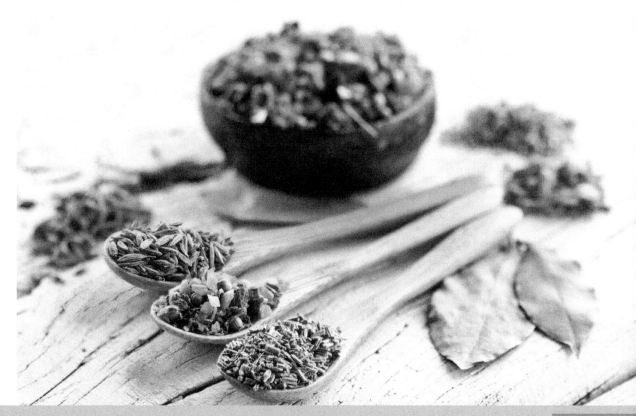

GARDEN BLEND

Makes 1/3 cup

This zesty blend is a great accompaniment for soups, salads, vegetables, fish, meat and poultry.

RECOMMENDED ESSENTIAL OILS:

1 drop of dill oil

1 drop of basil oil

1 drop of thyme oil

1 drop of orange oil

1 drop of onion oil

1 drop of celery seed oil

1 drop of oregano oil

WHAT YOU WILL NEED:

2 tbsp. dill leaves (or 1 drop dill essential oil)

2 tbsp. basil leaves (or 1 drop basil essential oil)

2 tbsp. thyme leaves (or 1 drop thyme essential oil)

1/2 tsp. orange zest, dried (or 1 drop orange essential oil)

2 tbsp. onion powder (and 1 drop onion essential oil)

1 tsp. celery seed (or 1 drop celery seed essential oil)

1/8 tsp. black pepper

1 tsp. oregano leaves (or 1 drop oregano essential oil)

1 tsp. salt

WHAT TO DO:

1. Dry all the ingredients and process them finely.

2. Stir in the essential oils that you choose and allow the mixture to dry. Transfer to a container and store until use.

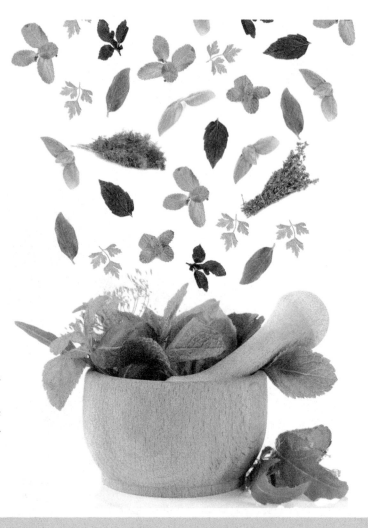

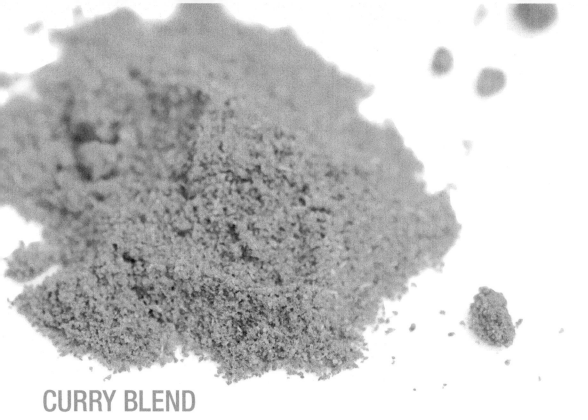

CURRY BLEND

Makes about 1/2 cup

This recipe brings a great flavor and an Indian style flair to soups, lamb, poultry and vegetables.

RECOMMENDED ESSENTIAL OILS:

1 drop of cumin oil
1 drop of turmeric oil

WHAT YOU WILL NEED:

2 tbsp. whole cumin seeds, toasted (and 1 drop cumin essential oil)

2 tbsp. whole cardamom seeds, toasted

2 tbsp. whole coriander seeds, toasted

1/4 cup ground turmeric (and 1 drop turmeric essential oil)

1 tbsp. dry mustard

1 tsp. cayenne pepper

1 tsp. salt

WHAT TO DO:

1. Start out by toasting the cardamom, cumin and coriander seeds.
2. In a bow, mix in the dry mustard, turmeric and cayenne pepper.
3. Stir in any essential oils you want to use and allow the mixture to dry if needed.
4. Place in a container. When you are ready to use, grind the mixture and add to the dish.

FLEUR DE SEL WITH THYME

This is the perfect salt to add to vegetables, meat and sweet desserts to capture the essence of French cooking.

RECOMMENDED ESSENTIAL OILS:

1 drop of thyme oil
1 drop of onion oil
1 drop of garlic oil

WHAT YOU WILL NEED:

Fleur de Sel
1 tsp. dried thyme (and 1 drop thyme essential oil)
1 tsp. onion powder (or 1 drop onion essential oil)
1 tsp. garlic powder (or 1 drop garlic essential oil)

WHAT TO DO:

1. Start with a bowl of fleur de sel and add in a pinch of dried thyme along the garlic and onion powders.
2. Stir in the essential oils using the toothpick method. Taste and add more thyme to taste. Allow to dry if needed and store in a container.

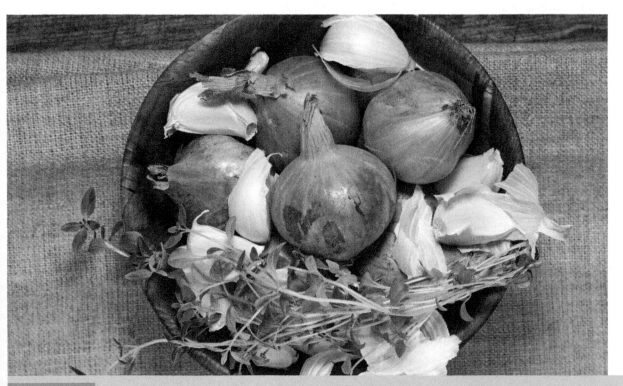

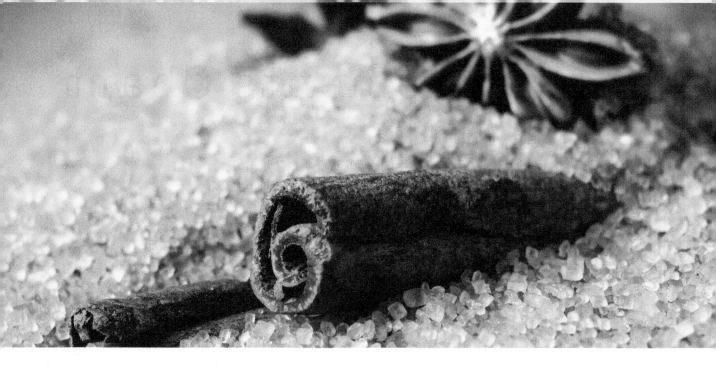

HOLIDAY SPICE

Makes about 1/8 cup

Time to make pumpkin and apple pies? Use this homemade spice to bring a little warmth and spice to your desserts.

RECOMMENDED ESSENTIAL OILS:

1 drop of cinnamon oil
1 drop of clove oil
1 drop of nutmeg oil
1 drop of ginger oil

WHAT YOU WILL NEED:

4 tsp. ground cinnamon (and 1 drop cinnamon essential oil)
2 tsp. ground ginger (or 1 drop ginger essential oil)
1 tsp. ground cloves (and 1 drop clove essential oil)
1/2 tsp. ground nutmeg (and 1 drop nutmeg essential oil)

WHAT TO DO:

1. Combine all of your dried ingredients in a bowl.
2. Mix in any essential oils you choose. Allow the mixture to dry if needed and store in a container.

Measurements Chart

LIQUID MEASUREMENTS

1 gallon = 4 quarts = 8 pints = 16 cups = 128 fluid ounces = 3.79 liters

1/2 gallon = 2 quarts = 4 pints = 8 cups = 64 fluid ounces = 1.89 liters

1/4 gallon = 1 quart = 2 pints = 4 cups = 32 fluid ounces = .95 liter

1/2 quart = 1 pint = 2 cups = 16 fluid ounces = .47 liter

1/4 quart = 1/2 pint = 1 cup = 8 fluid ounces = .24 liter

2 cups = 1 pint

4 cups = 1 quart

2 pints = 1 quart

4 quarts = 1 gallon

DRY MEASUREMENTS

1 cup = 16 tablespoons = 48 teaspoons = 237 ml

3/4 cup = 12 tablespoons = 36 teaspoons = 177 ml

2/3 cup = 10 2/3 tablespoons = 32 teaspoons = 158 ml

1/2 cup = 8 tablespoons = 24 teaspoons = 118 ml

1/3 cup = 5 1/3 tablespoons = 16 teaspoons = 79 ml

1/4 cup = 4 tablespoons = 12 teaspoons = 59 ml

1/8 cup = 2 tablespoons = 6 teaspoons = 30 ml

1 tablespoon = 3 teaspoons = 15 ml

1 teaspoon = 5 ml

1 gallon
- 4 quarts
- 8 pints
- 16 cups
- 128 ounces
- 3.8 liters

1 quart
- 2 pints
- 4 cups
- 32 ounces
- .95 liters

COOKING CONVERSION CHART

CAPACITY

1/5 teaspoon = 1 ml

1 teaspoon = 5 ml

1 tablespoon = 15 ml

1 fluid oz. = 30 ml

1/5 cup = 50 ml

1 cup = 240 ml

2 cups (1 pint) = 470 ml

4 cups (1 quart) = .95 liter

4 quarts (1 gallon) = 3.8 liters

1 tablespoon
- 3 teaspoons
- ½ fluid ounce
- 15 milliliters

WEIGHT

1 ounce = 28 grams

1 pound = 454 grams

COOKING MEASUREMENT EQUIVALENTS

16 tablespoons = 1 cup

12 tablespoons = 3/4 cup

10 tablespoons + 2 teaspoons = 2/3 cup

8 tablespoons = 1/2 cup

6 tablespoons = 3/8 cup

5 tablespoons + 1 teaspoon = 1/3 cup

4 tablespoons = 1/4 cup

2 tablespoons = 1/8 cup

2 tablespoons + 2 teaspoons = 1/6 cup

1 tablespoon = 1/16 cup

2 cups = 1 pint

2 pints = 1 quart

3 teaspoons = 1 tablespoon

48 teaspoons = 1 cup

1 pint

2 cups
16 ounces
480 milliliters

1 cup

8 ounces
240 milliliters

METRIC TO US COOKING CONVERSION CHART

1 ml = 1/5 teaspoon

5 ml = 1 teaspoon

15 ml = 1 tablespoon

30 ml = 1 fluid ounce

100 ml = 3.4 fluid ounces

240 ml = 1 cup

1 liter = 34 fluid ounces

1 liter = 4.2 cups

1 liter = 2.1 pints

1 liter = 1.06 quarts

1 liter = .26 gallon

WEIGHT

1 gram = .035 ounce

100 grams = 3.5 ounces

500 grams = 1.10 pounds

1 kilogram = 2.205 pounds

1 kilogram = 35 ounces

1/4 cup

4 tablespoons
12 teaspoons
2 ounces
60 milliliters

FOOD ADDITIVES LIST

Below you will find a compilation of all the botanicals that appear on the FDA's GRAS Food Additive list by a consensus of scientific opinion. Most of the items listed carry notations or restrictions like "flavorings for use in alcoholic beverages." The USDA Agricultural Research Center website reports that "many herbs are listed by the FDA because of their use in liqueurs and as components of natural flavorings prior to 1958, when the food additive regulations were written. However, alternative uses of the plant, such as flavoring water in an herbal tea, are presumably also safe, and the FDA has taken no action against any product on their list.

"Many herbal products fall into a 'gray area' of regulation. Around half of the herbs sold by the herb industry are not on the GRAS list, but are widely imported and sold for food use. Their omission from the list does not imply that they are not safe (for instance, barley and arrowroot are not GRAS food additives)."

This list is excerpted from the Code of Federal Regulations (CFR) Title 21 Parts 172, 182, 184, and 186. It is a listing of botanicals accepted by the FDA for food additive use, but does not include all plant derivatives; for instance, some plant gums, waxes and resins have not been included. All essential oils used for flavoring are included. In many cases species other than those listed are also used and may share the same common name.

Abbreviations used in this list are as follows:

Ext - Extracts
Fla - Flavorings
Oil - Oils
Olr - Oleoresins (total fat-soluble extract - oils, waxes, resins, volatile and fixed oils)
Pr - Less than 25 ppm prussic acid (a natural toxin)
Seas - Seasonings
Sp - Spice
SF - Safrole-free (a carcinogenic natural toxin)
TF - Thujone-free (another natural toxin)

Food Additives

A

Acacia (gum arabic) - EMUL/STAB, REG, Used as thickener, emulsifier, or stabilizer at =20% of alcoholic beverages-172.780, GRAS/FS, See Reg Part 135, Frozen Desserts; Part 169, Food Dressings and Flavorings; Part 169.179, Vanilla Pwd-184.1330

Allspice - SP/ESO, GRAS - 182.10 and 182.20

Allspice oil and oleoresin - ESO, GRAS - 182.20

Almond, bitter - ESO, GRAS, Free from prussic acid -182.20

Ambergris - MISC, GRAS

Ambrette (seed) - SP/ESO, GRAS - 182.10 and 182.20

Angelica (root, stem, seed) - SP/ESO, GRAS - 182.10 and 182.20

Angostura (cusparia bark) - ESO/SP, GRAS - 182.10 and 182.20

Anise, Star Anise - SP/ESO, GRAS

Apricot kernel (persic oil) - NAT, GRAS

Arnica flower extract - FL/ADJ, REG, GMP, In alcoholic beverages only - 172.510

Asafoetida - ESO, GRAS - 182.20

B

Balm (lemon balm) - SP/ESO, GRAS - 182.10 and 182.20

Balsam of Peru - ESO, GRAS - 182.20

Basil - ESO, GRAS - 182.20

Basil (bush and sweet) - SP, GRAS - 182.10

Bay, Bay leaves - SP/ESO, GRAS - 182.10 and 182.20

Bay (Myrcia Oil) - ESO, GRAS - 182.20

Bergamot (bergamot orange) - ESO, GRAS - 182.20

Bitter almond - ESO, GRAS, Free of prussic acid - 182.20

Bois de rose - ESO, GRAS - 182.20

C

Cacao - ESO, GRAS - 182.20

Cajeput - FL/ADJ, REG, GMP, In conjunction with flavors

Calamus, root, oil or extract - FLAV, ILL, Illegal in foods

Calendula - SP, GRAS - 182.10

Calumba root - FL/ADJ, REG, GMP - In alcoholic beverages only - 172.510

Camomile, camomile flowers English, Roman, German, Hungarian - SP/ESO, GRAS - 182.10 and 182.20

Camphor tree - FL/ADJ, REG, GMP, Comp of flavors - safrole free - 172.510

Cananga - ESO, GRAS - 182.20

Capsicum - SP/ESO, GRAS - 182.10 and 182.20

Caraway - SP/ESO, GRAS - 182.10 and 182.20

Caraway, black (black cumin) - SP, GRAS - 182.10

Cardamom (cardamon) - SP, GRAS - 182.10

Cardamom Oleoresin - ESO, GRAS, 182.20

Cardamom seed (cardamon) - ESO, GRAS - 182.20

Carob bean - ESO, GRAS - 182.20

Carob bean extract -ESO, GRAS -182.20

Carrot - ESO, GRAS - 182.20

Cascarilla bark - ESO, GRAS - 182.20

Cassia, cassia bark (Chinese, Padang or Batavia, Saigon) - SP/ESO, GRAS - 182.10 and 182.20

Cassie flowers - FL/ADJ, REG, GMP, In conjunction w/flavors - 172.510

Cayenne pepper - SP, GRAS - 182.10

Cedar, White (arborvitae) leaves and twigs - FL/ADJ, REG, GMP, Finished food thujone free, Used in conjunction with flavors - 172.510

Celery seed - SP/ESO, GRAS - 182.10 and 182.20

Centaury (centrurium) herb - FL/ADJ, REG, GMP, In alcoholic beverages only - 172.510

Chamomile Flower - SP, REG - 182.10

Chamomile Flower, English, Oil - ESO, REG - 182.20

Cherry-laurel leaves - FL/ADJ, REG, GMP, In conjunction w/flavors only; <25 ppm prussic acid - 172.510

Cherry, wild, bark - ESO, GRAS - 182.20

Chervil - ESO/SP/FLAV, GRAS - 182.10

Chervil extract - ESO, GRAS - 182.20

Chicory - ESO, GRAS - 182.20

Cinnamon and bark and leaf, Ceylon, Chinese, and Saigon -O/SP, GRAS, 182.10 and 182.20

Citronella - ESO, GRAS - 182.20

Citrus peels - ESO, GRAS - 182.20

Civet (zibeth, zibet, zibetum) - ESO, GRAS - 182.20

Clary (clary sage) - SP/ESO, GRAS - 182.10 and 182.20

Clove, bud, leaf, and stem - ESO, GRAS - 184.1257

Clover - SP/ESO, GRAS - 182.10 and 182.20

Cloves - SP, GRAS - 184.1257

Coca (decocainized) - ESO, GRAS - 182.20

Cocoa butter substitute from coconut oil, palm kernel oil or both - ESO, REG, Coating material for vitamins, citric acid, succinin acid and spices. In lieu of cocoa butter in sweets - 172.861

Coffee - ESO, GRAS - 182.20

Cola nut - ESO, GRAS - 182.20

Copaiba - FL/ADJ, REG, GMP, In conjunction w/flavors -172.510

Coriander - SP/ESO, GRAS - 182.10 and 182.20

Corn silk - ESO, GRAS - 182.20

Costus root - FL/ADJ, REG, GMP, In conjunction w/flavors -172.510

Coumarin - SY/FS, BAN, Any food containing coumarin added as such or as a constituent of tonka beans or tonka extract is adulterated.

Cumin (cummin) - SP/ESO, GRAS - 182.10 and 182.20

Cumin, black (black caraway) - SP, GRAS - 182.10

Curacao orange peel (orange, bitter, peel) - ESO, GRAS -182.20

Currant black, buds and leaves - FL/ADJ, REG, GMP, In conjunction w/flavors - 172.510

Cusparia bark - ESO, GRAS - 182.20

D

Dandelion, dandelion root - ESO, GRAS

Dandelion, fluid extract (Taraxacum spp.) - GRAS -182.20

Dill - SP/ESO, GRAS - 184.1282

Dill, Indian - FL/ADJ, REG, GMP, In conjunction w/flavors only - 172.510

Dog grass (quackgrass, triticum) - ESO, GRAS - 182.20

E

Elder Flowers - SP/ESO, GRAS - 182.20, 182.10

Estragole (or esdragol, estragon, esdragon, tarragon) -SP/ESO, GRAS - 182.20

Ethyl vanillin - SY/FL, GRAS/FS, Part 163, Chocolate and Cacao Pdts; Part 169, Vanilla Extract and Related Pdts - 182.60, 182.90

Eucalyptus globulus leaves - FL/ADJ, REG, GMP, In conjunction w/flavors - 172.510

Eugenol - SY/FL, GRAS - 184.1257

F

Fennel, common - SP, GRAS - 182.10

Fennel, sweet (Finochio, Florence) - SP/ESO, GRAS -182.10, 182.20

Fenugreek - SP/ESO, GRAS - 182.10, 182.20

Fir ("pine" and "balsam") needles and twigs - FL/ADJ, REG, GMP, In conjunction w/flavors - 172.510

G

Galanga (galangal root) - SP/ESO, GMP, GRAS - 182.10,

Galbanum - FL/ADJ, REG, GMP, In conjunction w/flavors only - 172.510

Garlic - SP/ESO, GRAS, GMP, 182.10, 182.20, 182.1317

Geranium - SP/FLAV/ESO, GRAS - 182.20

Geranium, East Indian or rose - ESO, GRAS - 182.20

Ginger - SP/ESO, GRAS - 182.10, 182.20

Glycoryrrhiza - SP/ESO, GRAS, See Reg - 184.1408

Glycyrrhizin, ammoniated - ESO, GRAS/FS, See Reg -184.1408

Grains of paradise - SP, GRAS, GMP - 182.10

Grapefruit - ESO, GRAS, GMP - 182.20

Guava - ESO, GRAS, GMP - 182.20

H

Hemlock needles and twigs - FL/ADJ, REG, GMP, In conjunction w/flavors only - 172.510

Hickory bark - ESO, GRAS, GMP - 182.20

Hop extract, modified - FLAV, REG, GMP, In beer - 172.560

Hops - ESO, GRAS, GMP - 182.20

Horehound (hoarhound) - SP/ESO, GRAS, GMP -182.10, 182.20

Horsemint - ESO, GRAS, GMP - 182.20

Horseradish - SP, GRAS, GMP - 182.10

Hyacinth Flowers - FL/ADJ, REG, GMP, In alcoholic beverages only - 172.510

Hyssop - SP/ESO, GRAS - 182.10, 182.20; Use in chicken and swine feeds

I

Immortelle - ESO, GRAS, GMP - 182.20

J

Jasmine - ESO, GRAS - 182.20

Juniper (berries) - ESO, GRAS - 182.20

K

Kola nut - ESO, GRAS, GMP - 182.20

L

Labdanum - FL/ADJ, REG, GMP, In conjunction w/flavors -172.510

Laurel berries, leaves - ESO, GRAS - 182.20

Lavandin - ESO, GRAS - 182.20

Lavender - SP/ESO, GRAS - 182.10; 182.20

Lavender, spike - ESO, GRAS - 182.20

Lemon, lemon peel - ESO, GRAS - 182.20

Lemon balm (See Balm) - ESO, GRAS - 182.20

Lemon grass - ESO, GRAS - 182.20

Lemon verbena - FL/ADJ, REG, GMP, In alcoholic beverages only - 172.510

Lime (citrus) - ESO, GRAS - 182.20

Linaloe wood - FL/ADJ, REG, GMP, In conjunction w/flavors - 172.510

Linden flowers - SP/ESO, GRAS - 182.20

Linden leaves - FL/ADJ, REG, GMP, In alcoholic beverages only - 172.510

Locust bean - ESO, GRAS - 182.20

Lovage - FL/ADJ, REG, GMP, In conjunction w/flavor -172.510

Lungmoss - FL/ADJ, REG, GMP, In conjunction w/flavors -172.510

Lupulin - ESO, GRAS - 182.20

M

Mace - SP/ESO, GRAS - 182.10

Malt (extract) - ESO, GRAS

Malt syrup (malt extract) - FLAV, GRAS, GMP -184.1445; nutrs in Part 133 (133.178, 133.179, 133.180); comp of color additive caramel - 73.85

Mandarin oil - ESO, GRAS - 182.20

Marigold, pot - SP, GRAS - 182.10

Marjoram, pot - SP, GRAS - 182.10

Marjoram, sweet - SP/ESO, GRAS - 182.10, 182.20

Mate - ESO, GRAS - 182.20

Melissa (see Balm) - ESO, GRAS - 182.20

Menthol - ESO, GRAS - 182.20

Mimosa (black wattle) flowers - FL/ADJ, REG, GMP, In conjunction w/flavors only - 172.510

Molasses (extract) - ESO, GRAS - 182.20

Mullein flowers - FL/ADJ, REG, GMP, In alcoholic beverages only - 172.510

Musk (tonquin musk) - MISC, GRAS - 182.50

Mustard, brown or black - SP, GRAS - 182.10

Mustard, white or yellow - SP, GRAS - 182.10

Myrrh - FL/ADJ, REG, GMP, In conjunction w/flavors only -172.510

Myrtle leaves - FL/ADJ, REG, GMP, In alcoholic beverages only - 172.510

N

Naringin - ESO, GRAS - 182.20

Neroli, bigarade - ESO, GRAS - 182.20

Nutmeg - ESO/SP, GRAS - 182.10

O

Oak moss - FL/ADJ, REG, GMP, Thujone free Comp of flavors - 172.510

Olibanum oil - FL/ADJ, REG, GMP, In conjunction w/flavors - 172.510

Onion - ESO, GRAS - 182.20

Opopanax - FL/ADJ, REG, GMP, In conjunction w/flavors 172.510

Orange bitter, flowers, peel - ESO, GRAS - 182.20

Orange sweet, leaf, flower, peel - ESO, GRAS - 182.20

Oregano (origanum, Mexican oregano, Mexican sage, origan) - SP, GRAS - 182.10

Origanum - ESO, GRAS - 182.20

Orris root -FL/ADJ, REG, GMP, In conjunction w/flavors -172.510

P

Palmarosa - ESO, GRAS - 182.20

Paprika - SP/ESO, GRAS - 182.10; color additive, GMP -73.340

Paprika oleoresin - ESO, GRAS - 182.20; color additive, GMP -73.345

Parsley - SP/ESO, GRAS - 182.20

Passion flower - FL/ADJ, REG, GMP - In conjunction w/flavors - 172.510

Patchouly - FL/ADJ, REG, GMP, In conjunction w/flavors -172.510

Peach kernel (persic oil) - NAT, SP/FL/ADJ, GRAS -182.40

Peach leaves - FL/ADJ, REG, GMP, In alcoholic beverages only, <25 ppm prussic acid in the flavor - 172.510

Peanut oil - GRAS, GMP, substance migrating from cotton in dried food pkg - 182.70

Pennyroyal (American) - FL/ADJ, REG, GMP, In conjunction w/flavors - 172.510

Pennyroyal (European) - FL/ADJ, REG, GMP, In conjunction w/flavors - 172.510

Pepper, black, white - SP/ESO, GRAS - 182.10, 182.20

Pepper, cayenne, red - SP, GRAS - 182.10

Peppermint - SP/ESO, GRAS - 182.10, 182.20

Persic oil (see apricot/peach kernel oil) - NAT, SP/FL/ADJ, GRAS - 182.40

Peruvian balsam - ESO, GRAS - 182.20

Petigrain (citrus aurantium) lemon, mandarin, or tangerine - ESO, GRAS - 182.20

Pimenta oil, pimenta leaf - ESO, GRAS - 182.20

Pine, dwarf, needles and twigs - FL/ADJ, REG, GMP, In conjunction w/flavors - 172.510

Pine, scotch, needles and twigs - FL/ADJ, REG, GMP, In conjunction w/flavors - 172.510

Pine, white, bark - FL/ADJ, REG, GMP, In alcoholic beverages only - 172.510

Pine, white oil - FL/ADJ, REG, GMP, In conjunction w/flavors - 172.510

Pipsissewa leaves - ESO, GRAS - 182.20

Pomegranate - ESO, GRAS - 182.20

Poplar buds - FL/ADJ, REG, GMP, In alcoholic beverages only - 172.510

Poppy seed - SP, GRAS - 182.10

Pot marigold - SP, GRAS - 182.10

Pot marjoram - SP, GRAS - 182.10

Prickly ash bark - ESO, GRAS - 182.20

Q

Quebracho bark - FL/ADJ, REG, GMP, In conjunction w/flavors - 172.510

Quillaia (soapbark) - FL/ADJ, REG, GMP, In conjunction w/flavors - 172.510

Quince seed - NAT, GRAS - 182.40

R

Rose absolute (otto of roses, attar of roses) - ESO, GRAS - 182.20

Rose buds, flowers, fruit (hips), leaves - ESO, GRAS

Rose geranium - ESO, GRAS - 182.20

Rosemary - SP/ESO, GRAS - 182.10, 182.20

Rue - SP/ESO, GRAS, < 2 ppm - 184.1698

Rue, oil - FL/ADJ, GRAS, See REG - 184.1699

S

Saffron - SP/ESO, GRAS - 182.10, 182.20 - Not permitted in standardized mayonnaise (169.140) or salad dressing (169.150); Color additive - 73.500

Sage, Greek - ESO/SP, GRAS - 182.10, 182.20

Sage, Spanish - SP, GRAS - 182.20

St. John's bread - ESO, GRAS - 182.20

St. Johnswort leaves, flowers and caulis - FL/ADJ, REG, GMP - In alcoholic beverages only, Hypericin-free alcohol distillate form only - 172.510

Sandalwood, white (yellow or East Indian), red -FL/ADJ, REG, GMP - In conjunction w/ flavors - 172.510

Sarsaparilla - FL/ADJ, REG, GMP, Natural flavor -172.510

Sassafras extract, safrole free - FLAV, REG, GMP -172.580

Sassafras leaves - FLAV/ADJ, REG, GMP, Must be safrole free - 172.510

Savory, winter or summer - SP/ESO, GRAS - 182.10,

Schinus molle - ESO, GRAS - 182.20

Senna, Alexandria - FL/ADJ, REG, GMP, In conjunction w/flavors - 172.510

Sesame - SP, GRAS - 182.10

Sloe berries (blackthorn berries) - ESO, GRAS - 182.20

Snakeroot, Canadian (wild ginger) - FL/ADJ, REG, GMP, In conjunction w/flavors - 172.510

Spearmint - SP/ESO, GRAS - 182.10, 182.20

Spike lavender - ESO, GRAS - 182.20

Spruce needles and twigs - FL/ADJ, REG, GMP, In conjunction w/flavors only - 172.510

Star anise - SP, GRAS - 182.10

Storax, or styrax - FL/ADJ, REG, GMP, In conjunction w/flavors only - 172.510

T

Tagetes (marigold) oil - FL/ADJ, REG, GMP, As oil only -172.510

Tamarind - ESO, GRAS - 182.20

Tangerine - ESO, GRAS - 182.20

Tannic acid - ESO, GRAS; NAT/FL/ADJ, GRAS, See REG, < .01% Baked Goods and Baking Mixes; < .015% - Alc bevs.; < .005% - Nonalc bevs.; < .04% - Froz dairy desserts and soft candy; 0.013% - Hard Candy; < 0.001% - Meat prods -184.1097; REG, In rendered animal fat - See 9 CFR 318.7

Tansy - FL/ADJ, REG, GMP, In alcoholic beverages only; Finished bev thujone free - 172.510

Tarragon - SP/ESO, GRAS - 182.10, 182.20

Tea - ESO, GRAS - 182.20

Thistle, blessed (holy thistle) - FL/ADJ, REG, GMP, In alcoholic beverages only - 172.510

Thyme, White Thyme - SP/ESO, GRAS - 182.10, 182.20

Thyme, wild or creeping - SP/FLAV/ESO, GRAS - 182.10, 182.20

Thymus capitatus (Spanish origanum) - FL/ADJ, REG, GMP, In conjunction w/flavors - 172.510

Tolu, Balsam, extract ands gum - FL/ADJ, REG, GMP, In conjunction w/flavors - 172.510

Tonka extract - SY/FL, BAN - See "Coumarin" - 189.130

Triticum (see dog grass) - ESO, GRAS - 182.20

Tuberose - ESO, GRAS - 182.20

Turmeric - SP/ESO, GRAS, Not permitted in standardized mayonnaise (169.140) and salad dressing (169.150) - 182.20

U

V

Valerian rhizome and roots - FL/ADJ, REG, GMP, In conjunction w/flavors - 172.510

Vanilla - FLAV, GRAS/FS Cacao Prods - Part 163; Food Flavorings - Part 169; SP/ESO, GRAS - 182. 10, 182.20

Vanillin - SYN/FL, GRAS/FS - Cacao Prods - Part 163; Food Flavorings - Part 169; GRAS - 182.60; Migr to food from paper and paperboard prods - 182.90

Vetiver - FL/ADJ, REG, GMP, In alcoholic beverages only - 172.510

Violet flowers and leaves - ESO, GRAS - 182.20

Violet leaves absolute - ESO, GRAS - 182.20

W

Walnut husks, leaves and green nuts - FL/ADJ, REG, GMP, In conjunction w/flavors - 172.510

Wild Cherry bark - ESO, GRAS - 182.20

X

Y

Yarrow - FL/ADJ, REG, GMP, In beverages only, finished beverages Thujone free - 172.510

Ylang-ylang - ESO, GRAS - 182.20

Yucca, Joshua-tree - FL/ADJ, REG, GMP, In conjunction w/flavors - 172.510

Yucca, Mohave - FL/ADJ, REG, GMP, In conjunction w/flavors - 172.510

Z

Zedoary - SP, GRAS - 182.10

Zedoary bark - ESO, GRAS - 182.20

OTHER BOOKS BY REBECCA PARK TOTILO

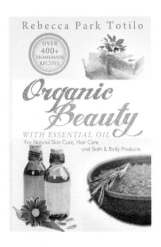

Organic Beauty With Essential Oil: Over 400+ Homemade Recipes for Natural Skin Care, Hair Care and Bath & Body Products

Sweep aside all those harmful chemically-based cosmetics and make your own organic bath and body products at home with the magic of potent essential oils! In this book, you'll find a luxurious array of over 400 Eco-friendly recipes that call for breathtaking fragrances and soothing, rich organic ingredients satisfying you head to toe. Included you'll find helpful can have the confidence knowing which essential oil to use and how much when creating your own body scrub, lip butter, or lotion bar! Discover how easy it is to make bath treats like fragrant shower gels, dreamy bubble baths, luscious creams and lotions, deep cleansing masks and facials for literally pennies using only a few essential oils and ingredients from your own kitchen with Organic Beauty with Essential Oil.

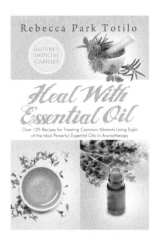

Heal With Essential Oil: Nature's Medicine Cabinet

Using essential oils drawn from nature's own medicine cabinet of flowers, trees, seeds and roots, man can tap into God's healing power to heal oneself from almost any pain. Find relief from many conditions and rejuvenate the body. With over 125 recipes, this practical guide will walk you through in the most easy-to-understand form how to treat common ailments with your essential oils for everyday living. Filled with practical advice on therapeutic blending of oils and safety, a directory of the most effective oils for common ailments and easy to follow remedies chart , and prescriptive blends for aches, pains and sicknesses.

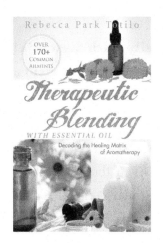

Therapeutic Blending With Essential Oil: Decoding the Healing Matrix of Aromatherapy

Therapeutic Blending With Essential Oil unlocks the healing power of essential oils and guides you through the intricate matrix of aromatherapy, with a compilation of over 170 common ailments.

Discover how to properly formulate a blend for any physical or emotional symptom with easy to follow customizable recipes. Now, you can make your own personalized massage oils, hand and body lotions, bath gels, compresses, salve ointments, smelling salts, nasal inhalers and more. This exhaustive guide takes all the guesswork out of blending essential oils from how many drops to include in a blend, to working with and measuring thick oils, to how often to apply it for acute or chronic conditions. It also shows you how to create a single blend for multiple conditions. Even if you run out of oil for a favorite recipe, this book shows you how to substitute it with another oil.

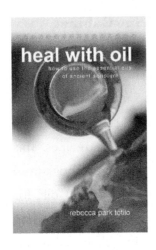

Heal With Oil: How to Use the Essential Oils of Ancient Scripture

God has provided a natural remedy to our Healthcare crisis - essential oils extracted from plants and trees. In this practical guide, Rebecca instructs believers on how to use the twelve healing oils mentioned in Holy Scriptures for healing and restoration of the body. Learn about the hidden treasures of the Levitical Priests and what the pharmaceutical companies don't want you to know. Book includes practical advice on blending oils and safety, a directory of properties for twelve oils from the Bible and special blends for the bath and personal care. Tons of recipes for beauty, health and emotional well-being.

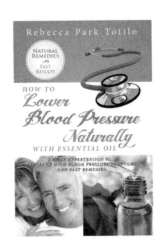

How to Lower Blood Pressure Naturally with Essential Oil: What Hypertension Is, Causes of High Pressure Symptoms and Fast Remedies

One out of three adults have it, and another one-third don't realize it. Oftentimes, it goes undetected for years. Even those who take multiple medications for it still don't have it under control. It's no secret -- high blood pressure is rampant in America.

High blood pressure, or hypertension, has become a household term. Between balancing meds and monitoring diets though, are the true causes -- and best treatments -- hidden in the shadows? In How to Lower Blood Pressure Naturally With Essential Oil, Rebecca Park Totilo sheds light on what high blood pressure is, the causes and symptoms of high blood pressure, and which essential oils regulate blood pressure and how to use essential oils as a natural, alternative method. Included within the pages of this book are simple blending techniques, dilution charts, and a wide variety of recipes for everyday use such as the Heart Plus Roll-On Blend and the Love My

Heart Massage Oil. Get creative with the basic blend recipes and discover your new favorite "medication." With no side effects and no prescription necessary, essential oils offer a healthy aromatic and therapeutic option for controlling your blood pressure.

This informative book will bust the myths of "questionable" oils, teach you how to make simple topical applications and inhalation methods, learn how to blend by "notes" to make super-easy recipes, examine numerous essential oil profiles and their common uses and reveal the health benefits of carrier oils.

Anoint With Oil

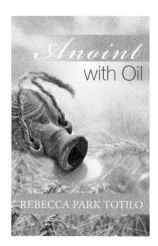

If you were taught by church leaders that anointing with oil ceased during the Old Testament times, or that it is simply "symbolic" and has no power or significance today, you may be missing beauty and depth in your spiritual journey. Anointing with oil brings real benefits into your life, such as promotion, discernment, sensitivity, fruitfulness, and declaration.

In Anoint With Oil, Rebecca Park Totilo shares an aromatic and sacred expedition through the scriptures, showing the purpose of anointing with oil, the methods used in the Bible and their symbolism, the ingredients of the holy anointing oil, and the uses of essential oils mentioned in the Old and New Testaments. Discover new scents within these pages and find out why the right ear, right thumb, and right big toe are used, what the mysterious fifth ingredient of the holy anointing oil is, which oils Jesus anointed with, who can perform an anointing ritual, and how you can benefit from anointing with oil.

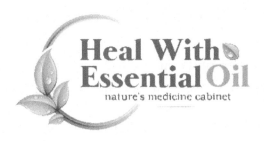

For other books, DVDs, and essential oils products, please visit our website:

http://HealWithEssentialOil.com

For e-mail correspondence, please write:

info@healwithessentialoil.com

For snail mail correspondence:

Heal With Essential Oil
P.O. Box 60044
St. Petersburg, FL 33784

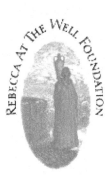

For More information about our teaching CDs, Books, and DVDs, please visit our website:

http://RATW.org

For e-mail correspondence, please write:

becca@rebeccaatthewall.org

For snail mail correspondence:

Rebecca at the Well Foundation
PO Box 60044
Saint Petersburg, FL 33784

CPSIA information can be obtained at www.ICGtesting.com
Printed in the USA
LVOW05s1922290315

432408LV00001B/1/P